PRAISE FROM AROUND THE GLOBE

"By emphasizing the whole food, plant-based diet as mankind's natural food, the authors of this book have deepened our understanding and our belief. I am convinced that this book will bring closer the day when cancer specialists the world over will wake up and realize that a new, effective treatment against cancer now exists and is ready for use."--**John Kelly, MD**, Dublin, Ireland, Author, *Stop Feeding Your Cancer*

"The big picture consequences of our food choices are not well known, even by beloved and well-meaning physicians. They, their patients and anyone interested in achieving optimal health will benefit greatly from this strikingly comprehensive, yet extraordinarily concise guide."--**Anne Ledbetter**, EdD, Director of Education, *T. Colin Campbell Center for Nutrition Studies*

"As a health and medical specialist, to me the 4Leaf Survey is a highly instructive and practical motivational tool, one I offer daily to most of my patients, from babies just starting solids--to the elderly. In my practice, I wouldn't be without it. The "4Leaf Guide to Vibrant Health" is therefore a must read."--**John Green, MD**, Family Physician, Melbourne, Australia

"Using food as medicine must become the foundation of a transformed and sustainable healthcare system, ushering in sustainable human health and a sustainable world. This information-packed guide is just what the doctor ordered--providing a powerful tool that medical professionals can use to confidently prescribe the 4Leaf lifestyle to their patients and clients."--**Susan Benigas**, Founder, The Plantrician Project (Plantrician ... Executive Director of the American College of Lifes

"As a rural south Arkansas family physician, I am attempting to educate my patients on the benefits of a plant-based diet--and this book will be a tremendous help. I particularly enjoyed Dr. Graff's dialog with her patients and her poignant letter to our fellow doctors."--**James Sheppard, MD**, Family Physician, El Dorado, Arkansas

"Armed with great passion and integrity, no one is more committed to promoting the health of humans AND the environment than these two authors. And that passion shines brightly in this inspiring book--a practical and powerful guide to plant-based eating at just the right time." --**Nelson Campbell**, Director, *PlantPure Nation* (Find this powerful 2015 documentary at PlantPureNation.com.)

"The compact *4Leaf Guide* delivers much more than you might expect, HUGE on relevant information presented in a clear and definable way! Let it help shepherd you to a life filled with rich and vibrant health!"--**Rip Esselstyn**, Author, *Engine 2 Diet* and *My Beef with Meat*

"In addition to summarizing the primary health and environmental benefits of adopting a whole food, plant-based diet, Dr. Graff and J. Morris Hicks include motivational case histories, access to valuable support resources and easy-to-understand tips and strategies. This *4Leaf Guide* will prove to be a valuable resource on your journey to better health." --**John Axelson**, PhD, Professor of Psychology, College of the Holy Cross, Worcester, MA

"Such a nicely written and easy-to-follow guide to aid the clinician in educating their patients. This is the result of what can happen when a physician realizes that the most important health information they can pass along to their patients is not yet being taught in medical school."--**Ted Crawford**, Doctor of Osteopathy, Tucson, Arizona

"Even though it is not in my economic self-interest, I highly recommend the plan put forth in this amazing book to anyone who is interested in optimizing their own health, the health of our Earth, and the health of all the non-human species who share this beautiful blue and green planet with us. As an Interventional Radiologist who repairs damaged arteries with angioplasty and stents, I personally profit from the havoc that the modern industrial diet plays on our arteries and organs. If everyone were to eat this way, I would be out of a job! Fortunately, I have a lot of hobbies."--**Ted D. Barnett**, MD, Interventional Radiologist, Rochester, New York

"Simply fabulous. I couldn't stop reading it until I finished. Loved it."--**Sheryl Greenberg**, Founder, *Healthy You Network*, Tucson, Arizona

"The thesis of this book is simple—and it provides solid, fact-based reasons for its conclusion: that it is imperative for humans to get off the meat, egg and dairy drug. For me, 4Leaf also alludes to the petals of the four leaf clover, representing faith, hope, love and luck. Lucky people will find this book--ethical and wise people will take its message seriously."--**Philip Wollen**, former head of Citicorp, Australia; now a Humanitarian Philanthropist

4LEAF GUIDE
To Vibrant Health

Using the power of food to heal ourselves and our planet

Kerry Graff, MD
and
J. Morris Hicks
Author, *Healthy Eating, Healthy World*

Library of Congress Control Number: 2015907036
CreateSpace Independent Publishing Platform
North Charleston, SC

ISBN-10: 1507613415
ISBN-13: 978-1507613412

Printed in the United States of America

4Leaf Global, LLC (a Connecticut company)
www.4leafglobal.com
Send feedback to info@4leafglobal.com

The publishers and authors of this book are not rendering professional advice or services for the individual reader. The ideas, procedures and suggestions in this book are not intended as a substitute for counseling with a physician. All matters of health require medical supervision. The publishers and authors shall not be liable or responsible for any loss or damage allegedly arising from any information or suggestion in this book.

CAUTION. Eating the 4Leaf way (described throughout this book) may quickly decrease your need for medications. You should tell your physician what you're doing. If he/she is not familiar with, or skeptical of, this eating style, please direct him or her to plantrician.org and nutritionstudies.org.

DEDICATION

To all of the innocent victims of humanity's collective
failure to follow nature's eating plan for our species

ACKNOWLEDGEMENTS

First, we would like to acknowledge the world-changing, breakthrough work of Cornell nutritional scientist, T. Colin Campbell, PhD and Cleveland Clinic physician, Caldwell Esselstyn, Jr., MD. Their courageous initiatives not only paved the way for the global plant-based movement that is happening today but also inspired the filming of the powerful *Forks Over Knives* documentary that facilitated the meeting of this book's two authors.

We also thank many other brave medical and dietary pioneers who have played a crucial role in this movement: Dean Ornish, Neal Barnard, John McDougall, Alan Goldhamer, Joel Fuhrman, Max Gerson, John Kelly, Michael Klaper, Nathan Pritikin, Herbert Shelton, Hans Diehl and Roy Swank.

Additionally, we are indebted to the great thinkers and environmentalists whose critical work has been instrumental in helping us better understand the "big picture" consequences of what we choose to eat: John Robbins, Howard Lyman, Robert Goodland, Jeff Anhang, Doug Lisle, Richard Oppenlander, Lester Brown and Stephen Emmott.

Finally, we acknowledge the ongoing dedication and active support of our 4Leaf team members: Kristin Keyes, Justine Robertson, Lisa Hicks and Jason Stanfield Hicks, the first person to use 4Leaf materials in promoting health.

TABLE OF CONTENTS

TABLE OF CONTENTS

INTRODUCTION

This *4Leaf Guide* contains everything you need to get started down the pathway to vibrant health. It also addresses what is arguably the most important issue in the history of humankind—our food choices in the 21st century. In the pages ahead, you'll learn all about why that issue is so important and why you should be eating a more optimal diet, for reasons that go far beyond your own health.

In the first chapter, Dr. Graff tells the gripping story of her own enlightenment when it comes to the power of food to cause or cure disease. She then explains how she leveraged her newly gained knowledge to begin the joyful process of "making good" on the incredible failures of her profession, which treats patients with pills and procedures while ignoring the huge role of diet in disease. In later chapters, Dr. Graff grants you a rare peek inside the physician's office as she gently leads her patients down the pathway to vibrant health.

This book introduces you to the simple 4Leaf approach to eating—an approach that promotes health for ourselves and for our planet. We will help you figure out what you ARE going to eat, rather than just what you should try to avoid. We will guide you in getting all the unhealthy stuff out of your kitchen and will provide tips to remember while shopping and eating out. We'll also provide some starter recipes and steer you to some great resources for many more.

Most of the chapters are less than five pages with descriptive titles so that you'll have no trouble finding what you need. In addition to gaining valuable tips for integrating this healthy way of eating into your busy lifestyle, you'll also learn how to deal with the plethora of questions, criticisms and unsolicited advice you'll be receiving from your friends, family and colleagues--as many of them may think that you have lost your mind.

Throughout the book, we hope to inspire you with a few success stories as told by Dr. Kerry Graff. Finally, you will gain an additional understanding by reading the Epilog by J. Morris Hicks, as he chronicles how we got into such a mess in the first place--a mess that includes staggering personal and global consequences of our poor dietary choices.

Looking for something specific? You can likely find what you need by just glancing at the table of contents. After completing this book, if there's anything you think that we may have missed, we encourage you to visit our website at 4leafprogram.com.

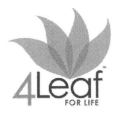

Promoting Vibrant Health.
For Ourselves. For Our Planet

1

PHYSICIAN HEAL THYSELF THEN OTHERS

By Dr. Kerry Graff

After almost twenty years of practicing medicine, I have Theresa Butler to thank for opening my eyes to the incredible failures of my profession. She was an elderly patient who came to see me for severe depression and anxiety. Her husband had died from colon cancer and I thought that might have been the trigger for her symptoms. It wasn't. Instead, she told me about her alcoholic son, Bobby, who still lived with her.

Bobby worked odd jobs a few hours a week and spent most of the little he earned on booze. Theresa paid all the bills, bought the groceries, prepared the meals and did all the housekeeping. In exchange, Bobby got drunk and beat her. Theresa had been seeing a counselor who set up a family meeting to intervene and get Bobby out of the house. She was so down and so anxious that she could barely function. I started her on an antidepressant and some anxiety medication to help.

On her next visit with me a few weeks later, she was smiling and much more relaxed. The family meeting had gone as planned and her son had been evicted. However, Theresa felt so much better from the medications I had prescribed, that she let Bobby move back in, confident that she could cope with his drunken aggression now that she had medication to "treat her anxiety."

That was the pivotal moment of my medical career, as I suddenly realized that by medicating patients, I was enabling them to continue the same destructive behaviors that caused their symptoms in the first place. That did not feel good--at all. In fact, I was sick to my stomach when I realized how often in my career as a family physician, I had treated someone for depression, fully intending to help them, but in reality, making it just bearable enough for them to stay in a bad relationship or a bad job.

Then it hit me. I was no different from Theresa Butler. I had been on antidepressants for twenty years but had not addressed what was making me so depressed in the first place! The medication kept me from jumping off a bridge, but made me too tired to actually change my situation.

I had not been listening to what my body was trying to tell me. Pain, whether physical or emotional, is information. It tells you "Something is wrong" or "Don't do that." It is uncomfortable for a reason--to get you to make a change! Medication was enabling me to stay in a situation that my body was clearly telling me wasn't healthy for me. Finally ready to listen, I stopped my antidepressant and it quickly became obvious what I needed to do. Honestly, it didn't even feel that there was a choice.

After the Theresa Butler incident, I was beginning to see a few trees in the forest, but I didn't start to see the whole forest of knowledge until I watched *Forks Over Knives*, the powerful documentary (featuring Dr. T. Colin Campbell and Dr. Caldwell Esselstyn) that presented the research behind the conclusion that we are killing ourselves with what we eat.

Oh God, another moment of profound nausea. If what they said was true, almost everything I had done as a physician for the past twenty years was just plain wrong. In essence, I had been letting people put their hands on a hot stove, then giving them pain medication to make it tolerable without telling them to "GET YOUR HANDS OFF THE #$%^%$ STOVE!"

Hoping the people in the movie were a bunch of veggie-loving quacks and I could just go back to doing business as usual, I checked out their research. I concluded that what they presented was true. As an experiment, I started eating the whole food, plant-based diet that they recommended. The effects were so stunning, so quick and so enormous, that I no longer had any trace of doubt.

Sugar levels—ALL normal when NONE had been normal prior. Reflux? Gone. Energy? Phenomenal. I no longer needed thyroid medication. And, without even trying, I lost the extra 25 pounds I was carrying! I felt and looked better than I had, well, EVER. Patients started asking what I was doing, and I started talking about this new way of eating and just never shut up.

In talking to patients about diet, I'd ask them to watch *Forks Over Knives*. Many would come back and say, "Wow. I get it. What I eat is making me sick. Now what do I do?" I needed something to help them bridge from WHAT they knew to HOW to do it.

Looking online for resources to help my patients, I found J. Morris Hicks' *4Leaf Survey* and his book, *Healthy Eating, Healthy World*. I emailed him to get permission (which he graciously gave) to use his survey and other 4Leaf materials as teaching tools for my patients.

I joke that my practice became the 4Leaf beta test site because virtually no one was using those 4Leaf materials prior to that. I have now used them hundreds of times and have seen amazing results in patients (and friends, and family!) who have embraced the 4Leaf way of eating-- simply striving to maximize the percentage of their daily calories from the healthiest of foods: whole plants.

I had spent the first half of my career putting patients on medications for various ills and then hounding them to take their pills to "stay healthy." Now, in an effort to undo the damage I had inadvertently caused while treating just the *symptoms* of disease, I have dedicated the second half of my career to focusing primarily on treating the *cause* of disease.

The US Center for Disease Control (CDC) estimates that 80% of the time, YOU have the power to prevent, reverse and even cure the diseases experienced in our western society by the lifestyle choices that you make. Seriously, YOU are so much more powerful than you think. And your doctor is so much less powerful than HE or SHE thinks!

It took me 44 years, seven abdominal surgeries, infertility (my kids were adopted), an episode of pulmonary edema from a "medical misadventure," 22 years of depression, treatment for hypothyroidism and reflux, developing pre-diabetes, and undergoing a mega-dollar workup for symptoms that looked life-threatening but turned out to be due to side effects from my antidepressant--before I figured out that the Standard American Diet and my lifestyle were making me sick.

Once I understood what to do, it took me less than three months to reclaim my health. Now it is my mission to help YOU reclaim yours. This *4Leaf Guide to Vibrant Health* will show you how.

Note: All patient names have been changed to protect confidentiality.

2

WHAT IS 4LEAF?

By J. Morris Hicks

4Leaf is an eating concept designed to make it easy for everyone to learn how to eat a near-optimal diet. Naturally, it all begins with the definition of the optimal diet for humans. In the interest of simplicity, I chose this statement by the Cornell professor who led the most comprehensive study of nutrition ever conducted. Here, he concisely summarizes his conclusions after a half-century career as a nutritional scientist:

> "The closer we get to eating a diet of whole, plant-based foods, the better off we will be."
>
> T. Colin Campbell, PhD, Nutritional Biochemistry

How simple is that? For a host of reasons that will be covered later, I am certain that the eating plan Mother Nature had in mind for the human species was one comprised of mostly whole plants. And we can help you get there with the information in the chapters ahead.

In this chart, we define six levels of eating, beginning with the least healthy Typical Western Diet. Each level is defined ONLY by the percent of its calories derived from whole, plant-based foods.

Unhealthful Diet Typical Western or SAD (Standard American Diet)	**Less than 10% of total calories from whole plants.** Containing some combination of meat, dairy, eggs, fish and/or highly-processed foods at almost every meal, this popular diet-style is associated with a plethora of serious health problems.
Better Than Most	**10% to 19% of calories from whole plants.** People at this level are actually trying to eat a healthier diet, but they need a better understanding of what promotes health.
1Leaf OVER 20%	**20% to 39% of calories from whole plants.** Although eating significantly more whole plants than the majority of folks, people at this level are not consuming enough of them to provide much protection against disease.
2Leaf OVER 40%	**40 to 59% of calories from whole plants.** Although eating 4-5 times more whole plants than most, people at this level are still falling short of ensuring long-term vibrant health.
3Leaf OVER 60%	**60 to 79% of calories from whole plants.** This group is deriving well over half of their total calories from health-promoting, whole, plant-based foods and is likely experiencing many of the benefits of healthy eating.
4Leaf OVER 80%	**Over 80% of calories from whole plants.** Currently representing a small minority of the population, these people tend to have trim bodies, vibrant health, lots of energy, take no medications, rarely have ANY disease and will likely live a long & healthy life.

The 4Leaf rule about fat content. Consumers of the Typical Western Diet (TWD) derive about 40% of their total calories from fat. Dr. Campbell and Dr. Esselstyn will tell you that the optimal percentage of fat in the diet is about 10%. Since achieving that number would be difficult for most people, we set the bar at 20%.

That means, to be a real 4Leaf-er, you not only need to derive over 80% of your total calories from whole plants, you also need to keep your percentage of fat below 20%. In order to do that, you may need to go easy on the following high fat content, whole plants: avocados, nuts, olives and seeds. Containing over 70% fat, these foods should be eaten in moderation only. The studies showing reversal of heart disease actually excluded these high-fat plant foods so, if you have heart disease, you may want to avoid them entirely.

The 4Leaf Survey. The 4Leaf approach to healthy eating was first introduced in my 2011 book, *Healthy Eating, Healthy World*. Later, in the spring of 2012, the 4Leaf Survey was introduced to help people estimate their own 4Leaf level of eating.

The survey (covered in Chapter 6) contains twelve simple multiple choice questions and can be completed in two or three minutes. The algorithm for scoring the survey and determining your estimated 4Leaf level was completed in 2014 after administering the survey over 40,000 times in the USA and abroad.

Daily Reporting Version of the survey. Unlike the standard 4Leaf Survey that is based on your recollection of your "average" eating habits, this version is based on what you actually ate on a particular day.

In Chapters 11 and 16, Dr. Graff explains the use of both of these surveys to one of her patients. Both versions of the 4Leaf Survey are included in the Appendix (A and B). Other 4Leaf materials can be found at 4leafprogram.com. They include the 4Leaf Chart and an extensive set of improvement tools. Additionally, there is a 4Leaf app in development.

In this book, we will do our best to help you achieve vibrant health by showing you how to eat at or near the 4Leaf level--getting over 80% of your calories from whole plants.

****

4Leaf is a registered trademark owned by 4Leaf Global, LLC, a Connecticut company. For information regarding use of this intellectual property, please visit our Policy Page at 4leafprogram.com.

4Leaf Global, LLC, was formed in 2015 with a mission of promoting the widespread adoption of whole food, plant-based eating throughout the world--for our own health and for the health of the ecosystem that sustains us.

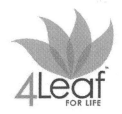

Promoting Vibrant Health.
For Ourselves. For Our Planet

3

WHY IS 4LEAF NEEDED?

By J. Morris Hicks

To help clear up the overwhelming CONFUSION in the developed world about what we should be eating.

A little history. Life began on our planet about four billion years ago. Humankind emerged as a species just 200,000 years ago--a mere blink in the eye of history. During those four billion years, there have been millions of different species of Earthlings, and Mother Nature had an eating plan for each one. Almost all of those millions of species have followed her plan to the letter, but not humans.

Why is that? We consider ourselves the smartest of all species, yet we still haven't figured out what we should be eating. As such, we now have hundreds, if not thousands, of different dietary theories--perpetuating the outrageous confusion that exists around what food choices are best for humans.

While some of those hundreds of eating plans are excellent, there are many that are extremely unhealthy. How is the average person supposed to sort through all of the hype and decide which are better and why? Here are 71 of those hundreds of dietary plans, from A to Z:

ATKINS, Best Bet, BEVERLY HILLS, Blood Type, BUDDHIST, Campbell Plan, CARNIVORE, China Study, CHIP, Colon Cancer, DASH, Diabetic, DUKAN, Eat to Live, EDENIC, Elemental, ENGINE2, Esselstyn Plan, FLEXITARIAN, Food Combining, FORKS OVER KNIVES DIET, Fruitarian, GLUTEN-FREE, Graham, GRAPEFRUIT, Hacker's, HALLELUJAH, Israeli Army, JENNY CRAIG, Junk Food, KANGATARIAN, Ketogenic, KOSHER, Lacto Vegetarian, LACTO-OVO VEGETARIAN, Locavore, MACROBIOTIC, Mcdougall Plan, MEDITERRANEAN, Neal Barnard's Program, NUTRI-SYSTEM, Nutritarian, OKINAWA, Omnivore, ORNISH PROGRAM, Ovo Vegetarian, PALEO, Pesca-Ovo-Lacto VEGETARIAN, Pescatarian, PRISON LOAF, Pritikin, RAW VEGAN, Scarsdale, SEARS, Shangri-La, SLIMMING WORLD, Slow-Carb, SONOMA, South Beach, STANDARD AMERICAN (SAD), Stillman, SUGAR BUSTERS, Vegan, VEGETARIAN, Warrior, WEIGHT WATCHERS, Typical Western Diet (TWD), WESTON A. PRICE, World of Wisdom, and ZONE.

Thirteen of the above eating plans would probably score at or near the 4Leaf level: McDougall Plan, Engine2 Diet, Ornish Program, Eat to Live, Pritikin, Dr. Esselstyn Plan, Raw Vegan, CHIP, Forks Over Knives, Campbell Plan, Fruitarian, Neal Barnard's Program and The China Study.

While the creators of those thirteen dietary plans may occasionally disagree on a few minor details, they would all agree that we should be getting the vast majority of our calories from whole plants. The simple 4Leaf Survey (in Chapter 6) makes it possible to quickly estimate your percentage of total calories derived from whole, plant-based foods--no matter which dietary regimen you are following.

Some of the 13 are considered extreme by many. I am referring specifically to Fruitarian and Raw Vegan. The world's healthiest populations eat mostly whole plants and include all of these food groups in their diets: vegetables, fruits, grains, beans and/or potatoes. And most disease reversal studies have focused on diets that include that full spectrum of whole, plant-based foods. Although Fruitarian and Raw Vegan diets, which are more limited, are very likely to have similarly positive effects on health and are certainly much healthier than the Standard American Diet, they have not undergone the same level of study.

Too much confusion. Many nights on the evening news, we hear about a new study that shows this and that about some obscure nutrient--a never ending flow of conflicting information that keeps the innocent public totally confused. It simply doesn't have to be so complicated. It's time for a healthy dose of clarity in an outrageously confusing world of dietary regimens. Our 4Leaf approach delivers that clarity.

That's because of the simplicity of 4Leaf, with each level of eating defined by the percentage of daily calories derived from whole plants. Any dietary regimen can be evaluated by its 4Leaf score, which compares it to the healthiest diet that is comprised of mostly whole plants.

When people are describing their vegan or vegetarian diets, I usually wonder what they are really eating. That's because they usually describe their diet by listing the things that they are NOT eating. And since what we ARE eating is so much more important, I simply ask them to please tell me their

4Leaf score. With that score in hand, I have a pretty good idea about the overall quality of their diet.

For a better understanding, I may ask them to send me a copy of their twelve multiple choice responses on the survey. With that information, I can tell them precisely how they might improve their score and their health. With this book, you will have all the information you need to determine that for yourself.

In addition, the 4Leaf Program allows for flexibility. While we would love for everyone to eat at the 4Leaf level, we realize that some folks are simply not willing to make that much change, regardless of the profound health and environmental benefits. It is up to each individual to choose how close they would like to get to an optimal diet comprised of mostly whole, plant-based foods.

The 4Leaf Survey and the other 4Leaf tools on our website were designed to help you measure your progress as you work to achieve your goal. The next chapter covers a plethora of reasons for why this way of eating makes so much sense.

4

WHY SHOULD WE EAT MOSTLY WHOLE PLANTS?

By J. Morris Hicks

Let's begin with a few nutrition basics. Humans fuel their bodies with three macronutrients: carbohydrates, fat and protein. We need some of all three to live, but we also need them in the right proportion to thrive.

In addition to macronutrients, we need vitamins, minerals, fiber and phytonutrients (naturally occurring chemical substances that help us fight off infection and cancer).

A varied, whole food, plant-based diet contains all of the above. In terms of calories, it contains roughly 80% carbohydrate, 10% fat, and 10% protein. It also contains tons of vitamins, minerals, fiber and phytonutrients. How do we know this way of eating is the healthiest diet for humans? Stay tuned.

The Typical Western Diet (TWD) or the Standard American Diet (SAD), with some combination of meat, dairy, eggs, fish and/or processed foods at almost every meal--provides a ratio of approximately 40% carbohydrates, 40% fat, and 20% protein. It provides very little fiber, vitamins, minerals or phytonutrients. What it does contain is a lot of fat and cholesterol (which clogs arteries) and animal protein. While you probably think that animal protein is a good thing, it turns our that it is associated with a multitude of diseases. More on that later.

As stated earlier, nature has a special eating plan for every species, but we have drifted far away from the plan that she had in mind for us. I could fill a one thousand page book with all of the information supporting why we should be eating mostly whole plants. But, for the sake of brevity, I offer you instead:

My Top 10 Reasons
For adopting a diet of mostly whole plants

1. The animal in nature whose DNA is nearly identical to humans (the gorilla) eats almost exclusively raw plants.

2. Observation of many healthy cultures like the Tarahumara of Mexico. Subsisting on mostly corn, squash and beans, they enjoy vibrant health, live very long lives and almost never have any of our chronic diseases.

3. Migrant studies. When members of those healthy cultures migrate to Chicago or Dallas and begin eating the toxic Standard American Diet (SAD), they begin to develop the same frequency of chronic diseases that we experience.

4. Disease reversal. The five medical doctors, featured in *Healthy Eating, Healthy World*, have leveraged the power of whole plants to successfully reverse heart disease and type 2 diabetes in over 90% of their cases.

5. Scientific Research. Dr. T. Colin Campbell of Cornell, author of *The China Study* and director of the largest epidemiological study in history, has validated the work of those above mentioned doctors with research that suggests that our consumption of animal protein (along with insufficient whole plants) is the primary driver of most of our chronic diseases.

6. Bill Clinton gave up his infamous burgers. Two of those five MDs and Dr. Campbell influenced him to adopt a whole food, plant-based diet in 2010. Love him or hate him, it's pretty big news when a former president of the United States, in order to reverse his heart disease, chooses a diet-style that has not yet been embraced by mainstream medicine.

7. Plants have plenty of protein. The strongest animals in the world (elephants, hippos and horses) eat almost exclusively raw plants. And they get plenty of protein, because nature put it there as part of their eating plan.

8. Kaiser Permanente. After considering the mountain of evidence, our nation's largest healthcare provider concluded that a whole food, plant-based diet is best for human health. In their 2013 Spring Journal, they reported: "Physicians should consider recommending a plant-based diet to all their patients; discouraging meats, dairy products, and eggs as well as all refined/processed foods."

9. Albert Einstein figured it out. He concluded: "Nothing will benefit human health and increase chances of survival for life on Earth as much as the evolution to a vegetarian diet."

10. The United Nations thinks it's vital. As reported in June 2010: "A global shift to a vegan diet is vital to save the world from hunger, fuel poverty and the worst impacts of climate change."

Notice in the last two reasons above that we start to widen our view, acknowledging that a whole food, plant-based diet also has a huge impact on the future of our society and our planet. Indeed, what we eat is the single most important topic in the history of humanity--because the future of humanity is riding on those food choices.

Without a doubt, the TWD/SAD style of eating is grossly unsustainable--not enough water or land, for starters. Our underground water reserves are being depleted at an astronomical rate in order to grow feed for livestock. And when there is no longer enough water to grow food for everyone, billions of people will die of starvation or from the violence that will ensue as people fight to survive.

The Bottom Line. A huge win-win awaits the Earth and all of her creatures when humankind begins a deliberate return to the natural diet for our species—one consisting of mostly whole, plant-based foods. You will learn more about that unprecedented *win-win* in the next chapter.

5

THE 4LEAF GLOBAL IMPACT

By J. Morris Hicks

In addition to you getting healthier, many great things happen when you start eating better. When you begin moving up the 4Leaf scale with your food choices, you'll be helping to improve far more about life on this planet than you ever imagined. Your own health is extremely important, but it's just the beginning.

When you start replacing meat, dairy, egg and fish calories with healthier, plant-based alternatives, you will be a part of the biggest win-win in the history of humanity:

- Win for your own health
- Win for our economy and cost of living
- Win for the health of our fragile ecosystem that sustains us
- Win for the future of our civilization and the long-term viability of the human species

In addition to the plethora of personal health benefits associated with better food choices, here is my top ten list of other great things we'll be doing for our world:

1. Cost of Healthcare. Standing at almost $3 trillion in just the USA, this economic nightmare is beginning to threaten our entire way of life in the developed world--where most of the unhealthy foods are eaten. Since the CDC estimates that 80% of our medical costs are lifestyle related with diet being a huge part, that $3 trillion number can be cut by more than $2 trillion when enough citizens begin eating at the 3Leaf or 4Leaf level. That helps everyone.

2. World Hunger. In a nutshell, there's simply not enough land and water in the world to feed everyone the Typical Western Diet. That's because, on average, the production of animal-based foods requires over ten times as much land, water and energy as do the same number of healthier, plant-based calories. If everyone ate the way we do in the USA, we'd need more than two planet Earths to feed us all--and we only have one.

3. Water Scarcity. This is our most urgent problem. One billion people don't have enough water today and it's getting worse all the time. Most of the water used by the average American goes to raise the livestock we consume, making it by far our single largest use (and waste) of water. It takes more water to produce one pound of beef than the average American uses to shower for an entire year! If you care about ending the world's water crisis, eat more plants!

4. Soil Erosion and Deforestation. Land is a finite resource and we're depleting it rapidly. Since 1970, we've destroyed some 30 million acres of rainforest a year--mostly for the raising of livestock. Each year, we lose an area of land the size of South Carolina to erosion, mostly due to the raising of billions of animals for our dinner tables.

5. Species Extinction. As a result of our actions in #4, we're destroying the natural habitats of hundreds of thousands of species. Every species in nature plays a role in the incredibly complex ecosystem that sustains us. Today, because of human activity (primarily the raising of livestock), the rate of species extinction is running at over 1,000 times the normal rate in nature. We humans are causing the biggest species extinction since the demise of the dinosaurs.

6. Dependence on fossil fuels. Another primary cause of climate change, our global consumption of fossil fuels has gone up every year since 1950--despite all the solar panels, electric cars and windmills that you see. The livestock industry uses massive amounts of fossil fuels to grow and transport animal feed and the livestock itself. Hence, one of the most powerful ways to actually start using less fossil fuel is to replace most of our animal-based calories with healthier, plant-based alternatives.

7. Climate Change. This is the elephant in the room and it exacerbates all the other problems we have. The U.N. reports that the raising of livestock generates more greenhouse gasses than all of transportation combined. Despite the fact that raising livestock is the leading cause of climate change, the largest environmental groups like Greenpeace and Sierra Club never mention it. Why not? Because being identified as "anti-meat" would hurt their fundraising efforts. Check out the documentary *Cowspiracy* to learn more about this infuriating issue.

8. Sustainability of our Civilization. If the alarming trends above are not reversed in the next ten years, many experts (Stephen Emmott, Lester Brown and others) agree that our civilization will ultimately collapse--well before the end of this century. We simply must learn to live in harmony with nature. Our future depends on it.

9. Sustainability of our Species. Who could not be concerned about this one? By definition, it has to be the most important issue in the 200,000-year history of humankind. And since all of the other issues threatening human survival on Earth will take many decades or centuries to fully address, that leaves only one viable pathway to the long-term sustainability of our species--a rapid move in the direction of a plant-based diet for humans. But that is not happening; in fact, it's the reverse. According to my extrapolation of United Nations Food & Agriculture Organization data, for every American or European moving toward eating more plants, there are 100 people in the developing world moving in the other direction.

10. Suffering of Animals. In addition to all of the above, what we're doing to the animals is abominable. Roughly 100 billion animals per year live a horrible life and suffer an awful death in this world so that we may eat their flesh. If you count the sea creatures, the number is over a trillion. And it's going up quickly as people in the developing world consume more meat, dairy, eggs and fish.

Are we in a hopeless situation? Not if we work together to influence billions of people throughout the world to simply begin to eat more plants. The good news is that this is the easiest, quickest and most powerful step we can take--and, as a bonus, it promotes our own health and it's delicious!

So let's get started. The win-win 4Leaf proposition is just too powerful to wait any longer. Begin by taking the 4Leaf Survey in the next chapter.

6

TAKE THE 4LEAF SURVEY

By J. Morris Hicks

The 4Leaf Survey is at the heart of the overall 4Leaf approach to healthy eating. By taking two minutes to answer 12 multiple-choice questions, you will get our best estimate regarding the percentage of your daily calories that are derived from the healthiest of foods: whole plants.

The scoring algorithm for the survey is based on "plus" points that can be earned in the first four questions and "negative" points that are earned in questions number 5 through 12.

If you take the survey online, your score will be computed automatically whereas, in Appendix A, we provide a simple way for you to compute your own score quickly. Also, by taking it manually, you will be able to see the exact number of points that you gained or lost on each question. Dr. Graff finds this feature particularly helpful in explaining the 4Leaf concept to her patients.

Could the 4Leaf Score be the next "vital sign" in medicine? The CDC estimates that poor diet is as harmful to health as is smoking. Yet, while smoking status is routinely assessed at every patient visit, evaluation of dietary health is neglected because a quick tool to assess its status has been lacking. Until now!

The simple 4Leaf Survey can be completed by patients in two or three minutes. The 4Leaf score generated serves as a dietary "vital sign," assessing the healthfulness of each patient's diet.

Take the 4Leaf Survey now. There are two ways that you can take the survey:

- **Online at 4leafsuvey.com**. A custom report, generated from your answers, will be emailed to you. That detailed report will show how you can improve your score AND, more importantly, your health.
- **Manually in Appendix A** on pages 151-153, where you can take the survey, score it yourself and be able to see exactly where you lost points and how you can improve your score.

Once you've taken the survey, proceed to the next chapter to learn more about your score and what it means.

7

WHAT DOES YOUR 4LEAF SCORE MEAN?

By Dr. Kerry Graff

The healthiest people on Earth get 80% or more of their calories from whole plant foods. Let's see how your diet compares. Now that you have your 4Leaf score, take a look at your *level of eating* below.

Unhealthful Diet. You are likely deriving less than 10% of your total calories from whole plant foods. This is the Typical Western Diet, also aptly known as SAD, or the Standard American Diet. You are eating some combination of meat, dairy, eggs, fish and/or highly processed foods at almost every meal. Currently, you are getting all of the health-damaging effects these foods cause, but you are NOT getting the health-promoting effects of whole, plant-based foods. Sadly, an estimated 65% of people living in western societies will score in this range.

Better Than Most. It is estimated that you are getting between 10-19% of your calories from whole plant foods. About 25% of people living in western societies will score in this range. People at this level are often trying to eat a healthier diet. They frequently say things like "I have given up red meat and am watching what I eat." Since about 65% of the western population scores in the "less-healthy" *Unhealthful Diet* range, you really are eating *better than most!* Unfortunately, however, you aren't even close to eating a diet that is likely to help you achieve vibrant health.

1Leaf. You are likely getting between 20-39% of your calories from whole plants. Approximately 10% of people living in western society will score in this range or better. You are eating significantly more whole plants than the majority of folks, which sounds great until you realize that you need to more than double your consumption of whole plants to be eating optimally!

2Leaf. It is estimated that you are getting between 40-59% of your calories from whole plant foods. We estimate that only 3% of the population is eating better than you. No doubt already working hard to eat a healthy diet, with a little "tweaking", you can easily move to the 4Leaf level and further raise your chances for a long, healthy life!

3Leaf. You are likely deriving between 60-79% of your calories from whole plants. Already eating a superior diet, you are likely experiencing many benefits from your healthy eating and are right on the verge of eating a 4Leaf diet.

4Leaf. Congratulations! It is estimated that you are deriving over 80% of your calories from whole plants and are among the healthiest eaters in the world. People in this group tend to have trim bodies, vibrant health, lots of energy, take no medications, almost never have ANY disease and will very likely live a long and healthy life.

You likely have questions about all of this. See next chapter.

8

FREQUENTLY ASKED QUESTIONS ABOUT THE 4LEAF SURVEY

By Dr. Kerry Graff

1. How accurate is the 4Leaf survey? You might be wondering how twelve multiple choice questions can be used to estimate your percentage of daily calories from whole plants. The key word is "estimate." As of this writing, our survey has been taken over 40,000 times since it was developed in April of 2012, with adjustments made to the algorithm to enhance its ability to estimate the 4Leaf score. No survey can be completely accurate with all the food options available to us, but ours works pretty well.

If you disagree with your results on our survey, try counting your actual calories on a typical day to determine your precise 4Leaf level. Simply divide your whole plant calories by your total calories consumed. Another thing you can do is to analyze your typical shopping cart. Add up the total calories from whole plants and divide by the grand total of ALL the calories in your cart.

2. Are fruitarians and raw vegans 4Leaf? Yes, they are, since they get over 80% of their calories from whole plants, even if they do not score at that level on the survey. And there are other exceptions. Some people just eat very few calories, yet over 80% of them are from whole plants.

If you're one of those people, then you're eating at the 4Leaf level, even if the survey indicates that you aren't. Again, the survey is just a tool to help people become more aware of how healthy (or unhealthy!) they are eating and to help them understand how they can improve their score-- and their health.

3. What is the difference between 4Leaf and vegetarian or vegan? When describing a diet-style, the "V" words only provide information about what you DON'T eat. Vegetarians don't eat animal flesh. Vegans don't eat animal flesh, dairy, eggs or any other animal products (like gelatin). 4Leaf, on the other hand, is about what you DO eat. The key to vibrant health (and the whole idea behind 4Leaf) is to get most of your calories from the healthiest of sources—whole plants. 4Leaf is about maximizing your consumption of whole plants (Questions 1-4) and minimizing the consumption of everything else. *That said, I do not recommend the consumption of ANY animal products.*

4. Why don't I get points for fruit or vegetable juice on my survey? First of all, juice is not a whole plant and the survey estimates your consumption of WHOLE plants. The good thing about drinking fruit or vegetable juice is that you ingest a ton of nutrients. But you also ingest a concentrated load of sugar and none of the fiber.

So juice is both good for you and not so good for you. Notice that, although juice doesn't count as positive points on the survey, it also doesn't count against your score.

5. Why don't I get points for whole wheat bread, cereal or pasta? While whole wheat bread and pasta are a heck of a lot better for you than the white flour versions, they are not as healthy as the unprocessed whole grains themselves. And, once again, they are NOT WHOLE PLANTS! This is another time when, although you don't get positive points for eating them, you don't get penalized either.

In the next chapter, I explain much more about the 4Leaf Survey and its uses.

4Leaf Tool Kit. Look for this at 4leafprogram.com. There you will find printer-friendly, one-page forms for the Standard 4Leaf Survey and the Daily Reporting Version. You will also have access to the expanded survey results for each 4Leaf level, and much more.

9

GOT MY SCORE; NOW WHAT?

By Dr. Kerry Graff

Are you surprised at how you scored? I sure was when I first took the survey! I thought I was eating a healthy diet but scored only at the *Better Than Most* level--not even 1leaf! If you didn't score very well, take heart. You have a lot of company.

Unless you are in the top 1% that scored at the 4Leaf level, you have what I call "improvement" opportunities. If you're already a *4Leaf-er*, you may want to stop reading this book right now and pass it along to someone who really needs it. Just kidding! Please continue reading so that you can fully explain to your friends and family how eating 4Leaf can help them--and our planet.

The 4Leaf scoring system is based on the ultra-simple concept of "plus" points for eating whole plants and "minus" points for just about everything else.

Take a look at your responses to questions 1 to 3 on the survey. If you did not score at least 12 points on each of these questions by eating three or more servings in each category, you will improve your health by increasing these types of foods in your diet. You will not only get more of the nutrients that help your body function, you will also naturally eat less of the foods that contribute to chronic disease.

Now take a look at your responses on questions 5 through 12. Where did you lose points? Cut back on, or better yet, eliminate those animal-based or highly processed foods (the oil, cream, milk, yogurt, cheese, eggs, meat, white flour and fish). Don't worry; you'll still be getting plenty of protein and calcium. More on that later.

Take breakfast for example. Let's say you usually eat an egg, ham and cheese sandwich on an English muffin. You just lost points for dairy, meat, egg and white flour. You didn't even get one positive point because 0% of the calories from your breakfast came from whole plant foods.

What if you ate oatmeal with fruit and a little almond milk instead? Over 90% of your calories would come from whole plant foods. (The almond milk isn't a whole plant, but it is plant-based and you won't use that much.)

Now think about lunch and dinner. What happens when you swap out your tuna fish on white bread and potato chips for a bowl of vegetable soup with beans or rice? Get the picture? When you swap out negative points for positive ones, you improve your score (and your health) fast!

What about that omega-3 question? Okay, I admit that it is sort of a trick question. If your answer was anything other than "Yes," you're probably thinking you need to consume a little fish or fish oil in order to get enough of this nutrient. You don't.

Here's the scoop. It is actually the ratio of omega-3 to omega-6 that is important. A diet with lots of animal-based and processed foods contains huge amounts of inflammation-causing omega-6 compared to small amounts of inflammation-calming omega-3.

With the ratio out of whack, we get sick. The ratio of omega-3 to omega-6 in plant-based foods is perfect without needing to add a thing. So if you are eating only plants, you don't need to specifically add any omega-3s by eating flax, hemp, or chia seeds or walnuts. That said, I love a few walnuts on my oatmeal in the morning. Yum!

A word on plant-based meat and cheese substitutes. I don't mean to unjustly criticize the latest generation of those plant-based analogues for meat, dairy, eggs and mayo; they do serve a purpose for some people, especially in the early stages. I just know that, for your health, a variety of whole, plant-based foods, still in nature's package, are your best bet.

Bottom Line. Embrace and nurture your healthy eating adventure. Find great recipes and learn to prepare some of the most delicious meals that you will ever eat. Avoid the temptation to establish your new routine around the processed plant-based substitutes for meats and cheeses. Trust me, you will come to LOVE the taste of fruits, vegetables and grains and you will also love how you look and feel!

So, should moving to this new diet-style be a gradual process or should you take the plunge and go all the way from the start? That's the question that I address in the next chapter.

10

BABY STEPS
OR ALL THE WAY?

By Dr. Kerry Graff

Okay, you have decided that you want to achieve vibrant health. Should you take baby steps and start out by adding a few fruits and vegetables to your diet and gradually work your way up the 4Leaf scale? Or should you jump into the deep end of the pool and start swimming with all you've got?

To answer that question, you may want to consider the following statements from these whole food, plant-based experts:

> **Dr. Dean Ornish**: "In our research, we learned that it is often easier for people to make comprehensive changes in diet and lifestyle than to make only moderate ones. At first, this may seem like a paradox, but it makes sense when you understand why. If you make only moderate changes in lifestyle--then you have the worst of both worlds. You feel deprived and hungry because you are not eating everything you want

and are used to, but you're not making changes big enough to feel that much better or to significantly affect your weight or how you feel, your cholesterol, blood pressure or heart disease."

Dr. John McDougall: "If you are sincere about making the change, do so with 100% of your effort. Many people feel that it would be easier for them to slide into this diet plan gradually. Unfortunately, we seldom manage to discard old ways and old established tastes unless 100% of our effort is devoted to the change and unless, from the beginning, we make a clear break from our old behavior. A smoker who cuts down to four cigarettes a day only goes through slow torture and rarely quits completely."

Dr. T. Colin Campbell: "Following this diet requires a radical shift in your thinking about food. It's more work to just do it halfway. If you plan for animal-based products, you'll eat them--and you'll almost certainly eat more than you should. You'll feel deprived. Instead of viewing your new food habit as being able to eat all the plant-based food you want, you'll be seeing it in terms of having to limit yourself, which is not conducive to staying on the diet long-term."

Dr. Caldwell Esselstyn sums up his advice on this subject in just two words: "Moderation kills."

While there are exceptions, the greater your commitment to the 4Leaf way of eating in the beginning, the greater the likelihood that your healthier eating habits will be permanent and that you will achieve and maintain the lifelong benefits of vibrant health that you seek.

In pursuit of vibrant health. 4Leaf is a simple, yet powerful, way to eat that will reward you for the rest of your life. It is well worth the effort to make 4Leaf a permanent lifestyle change in your pursuit of vibrant health. So how do you begin a permanent lifestyle change? It all begins with commitment.

By reading this book, you've already made a commitment-- to learn about the health-promoting, whole food, plant-based way of eating. Congratulations! After you have finished reading this book, I want you to make another commitment. Well, actually, I want you to make two.

> **Commitment 1: To 4Leaf in 4 weeks**. I want you to get to the 4leaf level of eating as quickly as possible, but I also understand that you have to learn a whole new way of thinking about food. For most people, that isn't going to happen overnight. You will need to learn new recipes and create new habits. So, although I recommend that you shift as rapidly as you can all the way to the 4leaf level, I suggest that you take no longer than four weeks to get there for all the reasons stated by the experts above.

> **Commitment 2: Eat 4Leaf for 4 months.** I strongly recommend that, once you get to the 4Leaf level of eating, you stick with it for at least four months. After that, you will look and feel so much better and the habits will be so ingrained, that you are likely to eat 4Leaf for the rest of your very long and healthy life.

Wiggle Room. I get it that nobody likes "all or nothing." While there's implied "wiggle room" in the 4Leaf formula (since you can reach the 4Leaf level with only 80% of your calories from whole plants), I recommend that you try to avoid ALL the foods that result in negative points in the survey for the duration of your commitment period.

Yup, I mean trying to avoid all meat, dairy, eggs, cheese, fish, sweets, salty snacks, white flour, sugars and oils. If you eat some cheese by mistake at a potluck dinner, it's not a big deal. In our society, these unhealthy foods are ubiquitous and nearly impossible to avoid entirely. The main point is that you don't "plan" to eat any of these foods during your all-important commitment period.

Baby Stepping. Although I don't recommend baby steps, I do acknowledge that some people have been successful at reaching the 4Leaf level after taking the leisurely route down the pathway to vibrant health. I also acknowledge that eating at the 2Leaf level for the rest of your life is much better for your health than eating at the *Unhealthful Diet* level for your likely shorter and sicker life.

But it is your life and, of course, it is your choice as to what level you aim for and how quickly you choose to get there. We really do (80% of the time, anyway) choose to be sick or healthy by the decisions we make every day. I hope that you choose the 4Leaf level of eating and that you will be rewarded with the very best health possible.

You're now ready to start figuring out what you ARE going to be eating for the next few months--and hopefully, for the rest of your life. You might be interested in how I explained this whole concept to one of my patients in the next chapter.

11

EXPLAINING
4LEAF TO MY PATIENTS

By Dr. Kerry Graff

I asked Tom Miller, a 52 year old patient who was a fitness fanatic with recurrent kidney stones, to come in to discuss findings on his CT scan, ordered by his urologist.

KG: "Tom, your CT scan didn't show any more kidney stones, but it did show a significant amount of plaque in your biggest artery, the aorta. Plaque is caused by cholesterol and fat clogging up blood vessels over time. Are you having any symptoms of leg or chest pain or reduced ability to exercise due to shortness of breath?"

TM: "Are you kidding me?! I eat a really healthy diet and exercise at least 3 days a week for a couple of hours. I quit smoking 25 years ago. I can't believe it--and no, I am not having any chest or leg pain or shortness of breath."

KG: "I know it must come as a shock when you feel like you are doing all the right things for your health. I got the results of the blood work you had drawn, though, and they weren't good. Your total cholesterol was 272, and although you have a high amount of the good cholesterol called HDL, your LDL, the bad cholesterol, was 177 when it should be below 130. Your triglycerides were also high at 222, when they should be under 150."

TM: "This has got to be genetic! I am doing everything right!"

KG: "It is possible that you are, but I'd like to go through a diet survey to see if there is a cause in your diet before we jump to medication."

Tom took the 4Leaf Survey and scored -7, only at the *Better Than Most* level. Despite eating lots of veggies and fruit, an estimated 80-90% of his calories were coming from animal products and processed foods rather than whole plant foods. What was he doing right? Eating three servings of fruits and vegetables a day and avoiding most processed foods.

Where did he go wrong? He thought that eating white meat and seafood was fine as long as he avoided red meat. He was also eating lots of dairy products, using a lot of olive oil, eating lots of eggs "for the protein," and drinking 4 glasses of red wine every night.

KG: "Tom, I'm not sure yet if you are one of the people who has a genetic problem with their cholesterol and need medication to get their levels down. I do know that even if you do have the genetic problem, eating cholesterol, which is present in animal products but not in plants, is like throwing gasoline on a fire. It just makes the problem worse. I'd like you to watch a documentary called *Forks Over Knives* to get an overview of why we think that eating mostly whole plants is the best diet for humans.

I have the DVD here that I can lend you or you can watch it on Netflix, if you have that. The diet they talk about in the movie, the one you just scored your diet against with the 4Leaf Survey, not only can prevent further plaque from forming, it can actually reverse it. Check out what Dr. Esselstyn did with the heart patients whom the Cleveland Clinic gave up on!"

TM: "Are you saying I'm a heart patient now?!"

KG: "Well, plaque deposits or atherosclerosis, is really a disease of the blood vessels and it isn't isolated to just one area. So it is likely that all of your vessels are affected. The good news is that you are very active physically and, despite that, haven't had symptoms yet. Let's keep it that way by changing your diet. Another plus is that this way of eating reduces formation of further kidney stones, which have given you a lot of grief through the years."

TM: "That would be great. My kidney stones have been miserable. I've had stents put in when the stones have blocked off my kidneys. But what I really don't want is a heart attack!"

KG: "You and I will work on more diet changes I'd like you to make over time, but for now, I'd like you to watch the documentary so you really understand why this diet works. And make the following changes until we regroup next week:

1. Stop eating all dairy.

2. Eat oatmeal (the kind that takes 5 minutes or more to cook) with some fruit in it rather than eggs for breakfast.

3. Use a plant based milk like almond or soy instead of cow's milk.

4. Eat soup for lunch rather than your turkey, cheese and mayo sandwich. Veggie soup with beans or rice would be good. Or black bean soup or a veggie chili.

5. Cut back to no more than two glasses of wine a day."

TM: "But why do I have to cut back on the alcohol? There's no cholesterol in wine, is there?"

KG: "No, there isn't. But triglycerides are a mixed molecule of fat AND sugar. And wine has a lot of sugar in it and so will raise triglycerides. The amount of alcohol you are drinking is hard on the liver too. If you are drinking because you are anxious, we should talk about other ways to manage your stress.

We've covered a lot today and you've certainly got some homework and a lot of thinking to do before our next visit in about a week. In the meantime, please call our office if you have any urgent questions."

****

If this 4Leaf Guide had been available at the time, I would've asked Tom to pay particular attention to the next chapter (and the referenced appendices) before our next visit.

12

GOING 4LEAF IN 4 WEEKS

By Dr. Kerry Graff

The truth is that you can transition to the 4Leaf level any way you want. When I work one-on-one with patients, I develop individualized plans based on their schedules and preferences. I start with changes that are pretty easy to make but that also have a big impact on the overall quality of that patient's diet. I find out what healthy foods they enjoy already and suggest they eat those foods more often, before having them move on to new recipes.

In the group classes I run, individualized coaching is just not possible and I need to be more structured. I have found that it is easiest to base the classes around transitioning each meal over the course of a month. The following is the basic plan (details in Appendix C) that I use for my classes:

Week 1--Planning stage. Figure out what your weekly plan will be for meal planning, food shopping and batch cooking. Decide what you want to eat for your routine breakfast and healthy snacks. Before the end of Week 1, get rid of all the unhealthy breakfast and snack foods.

Week 2--Breakfast and snacks. Enact your weekly plan for meal planning and shopping. Start eating a 4Leaf breakfast every day and healthy snacks. Track your progress using the 4Leaf Survey daily reporting version. Start thinking about some 4Leaf lunch options for the next week. Start stocking your pantry with healthy staples (oats, nuts, beans, grains like bulgur, brown rice, and quinoa, etc.)

Week 3--Lunch. Continue your plan for meal planning and shopping. Continue eating your 4Leaf breakfasts and snacks. Start batch cooking and eating a 4Leaf lunch every day as well. Continue to use the 4Leaf Survey to track your progress. Start thinking about what 4Leaf dinners you might want to have next week. By the end of week 3, get rid of the rest of the unhealthy foods in the house.

Week 4--Dinner. Continue your plan for meal planning, shopping and batch cooking. Continue eating your 4Leaf breakfasts, lunches and snacks and add in 4Leaf dinners. Continue to use the 4Leaf Survey to track how you are doing. You should be scoring at a 4Leaf level every day. If you are not, evaluate where you are scoring negative points or not scoring enough positive ones.

Next Step. Once you have finished reading this book and (hopefully!) have decided you want to go 4Leaf, decide if you want to develop your own plan or follow my weekly plan. It doesn't matter how you get to 4Leaf, just that you do!

Going 4Leaf Series in the Appendix

13

RECIPES ARE EVERYWHERE

By Dr. Kerry Graff

While this book contains a few recipes to get you started, Jim and I didn't put dozens of recipes in this little book. Here's why:

1. We wanted to keep this book inexpensive so that just about anyone who was interested could afford it. That meant keeping it small and in black and white. Recipes, on the other hand, are much more appealing with beautiful color pictures to inspire you.

2. Most people have at least one internet-enabled electronic device with a plethora of healthy recipes at their fingertips at all times. And many of them are free.

3. We think it's more valuable if we show you how to find or create hundreds of great recipes on your own. Remember the "teach a man to fish" tale?

Recipe Websites. We asked many of our plant-based eating friends for their favorite free recipe websites. Fourteen of those sites are listed here in alphabetical order.

1. 4LeafProgram.com
2. ChocolateCoveredKatie.com (desserts)
3. DrMcDougall.com
4. Engine2Diet.com
5. FatFreeVegan.com
6. ForksOverKnives.com (plus great app)
7. HappyHerbivore.com
8. NakedFoodMagazine.com
9. NutritionStudies.org
10. OhSheGlows.com
11. OneGreenPlanet.org
12. Peta.org/recipes
13. StraightUpFood.com
14. TheSimpleVeganista.blogspot.com

Cookbooks. Some of you will prefer to use an actual cookbook rather than a website or app. (As the daughter of two English teachers, I love books and cookbooks are no exception.) Here are some of our favorites, all of which are available at Amazon.

* *The China Study All Star Collection*, Leanne Campbell
* *The China Study Cookbook*, Leanne Campbell
* *Forks Over Knives The Cookbook*, Del Sroufe
* *The Happy Herbivore* (all of them), Lindsay Nixon
* *The Oh She Glows Cookbook*, Angela Liddon
* *PlantPure Nation Cookbook*, Kim Campbell
* *Straight From the Earth*, Myra and Marea Goodman
* *Thrive Energy Cookbook*, Brendan Brazier

The following aren't just *cookbooks* but do contain a lot of recipes, along with other great information on whole food, plant-based diets:

- *Engine 2 Diet* and *My Beef with Meat*, by Rip Esselstyn
- *Forks Over Knives, The Plant-based Way to Health*, Gene Stone
- *The Forks Over Knives Plan* An excellent book on how to transition to plant-based eating whose only flaw is not using the 4Leaf Survey tool! By Alona Pulde and Matthew Lederman
- *Prevent and Reverse Heart Disease*, by Caldwell Esselstyn

Note that some of the recipes on these sites or in the cookbooks will not score at the 4Leaf level, but they are a good place to start. Some of the recipes have oil, which we recommend you leave out. Some will contain whole grain but processed, plant-based foods, which we encourage you to use in moderation.

Create your own favorite recipes. One of Jim's favorite creations is his *Sailors Daily Oatmeal*. He figures if a single man with minimal cooking experience can create a recipe, anyone can. For more details about that recipe, see page 160 or visit Recipes at 4leafprogram.com.

Recipes in Appendix. Beginning with Appendix C on page 156, you will find a number of our favorite recipes in the *Going 4Leaf in 4 Weeks* series.

One more idea. Jim and I have found many great recipes at mainstream sources like the *New York Times*. Quite a few of their recipes can be tweaked a bit and quickly turned into a fairly healthy 3 or 4Leaf meal. We call this Meal Engineering 101: turning average meals into great-tasting, nutritious, health-promoting meals.

14

FOOD SHOPPING AND CONTRABAND

By J. Morris Hicks

I learned the word "contraband" while serving in the United States Coast Guard. It means "goods imported illegally." So, if you still have cheese in your refrigerator and beef in your freezer, you can now refer to those items as contraband--when it comes to 4Leaf eating.

Technically, you could score at the 4Leaf level and still eat a little contraband every now and then, but I'm going to try to help you learn to live happily ever after without those foods which do not contribute to your vibrant health.

Here's the deal with contraband and shopping for food: "If it goes into your shopping cart, it will end up in your stomach." First, we get the contraband out of the kitchen and next we work on not bringing anymore home.

Cleaning out your kitchen. As with your shopping cart, if you still have contraband in your kitchen, there's a good chance that it will end up in your stomach. So what do you do with it? Throw it all away?

No, but don't put it in your basement either. That would be a signal to your brain that this is a temporary way of eating. Not good to play tricks on your brain; rather, you want to do everything you can to maximize your chances for success by getting your subconscious brain acclimated to the 4Leaf mentality.

So what do you do with all that cheese, milk, yogurt, ice cream, canned meats, frozen meals with meat and dairy, frozen burgers, chicken, etc.? I recommend that you package them all up and give them away to charity, a neighbor, a friend or a family member.

My son Jason disagreed, saying that it would be unethical to give away food that you might now consider to be a form of poison. But, for me, I hate to see waste of any kind, and throwing away food that the majority of people think of as wholesome, is a huge waste.

Think of it this way. Whether you donate your meat and dairy products or not, the recipients will likely continue to eat them for a very long time. Or at least until they see your *before and after* pictures. By donating that food, you're just making sure that fewer animals have to suffer and die, in order to replace the edible food that you trashed.

Shopping for Groceries. The first thing you need to do is make a list of all the items that you will need to prepare the routine meals that you plan to eat at home. You should always have a list.

Another tip is to get most of your food from the fresh produce section and the section that has dried grains and legumes. While in those areas, you will not find a "Nutrition Facts" panel on most of the products. It's not needed for fresh whole plants, but is required for all packaged foods.

When buying processed food in a package, find the Nutrition Facts panel, which is usually on the back or the side of the package. Let's look at five things on this panel: Calories from Fat, Cholesterol, Sodium, Fiber and Sugars. Everything else is pretty much worthless.

Nutrition Facts

Serving Size 1 cup (228g)
Servings Per Container 2

Amount Per Serving

Calories 250   Calories from Fat 110

	% Daily Value*
Total Fat 12g	**18%**
Saturated Fat 3g	**15%**
Trans Fat 3g	
Cholesterol 30mg	**10%**
Sodium 470mg	**20%**
Total Carbohydrate 31g	**10%**
Dietary Fiber 0g	**0%**
Sugars 5g	
Protein 5g	

Vitamin A	**4%**
Vitamin C	**2%**
Calcium	**20%**
Iron	**4%**

* Percent Daily Values are based on a 2,000 calorie diet. Your Daily Values may be higher or lower depending on your calorie needs.

	Calories:	2,000	2,500
Total Fat	Less than	65g	80g
Sat Fat	Less than	20g	25g
Cholesterol	Less than	300mg	300mg
Sodium	Less than	2,400mg	2,400mg
Total Carbohydrate		300g	375g
Dietary Fiber		25g	30g

1. Calories from Fat. To compute the percentage fat, divide "Calories from fat" by total "Calories" per serving. Use your smartphone calculator if you must, but you can usually eyeball it and tell if the product is more than 20% fat. You can easily see that this product is over 40% fat (110/250 = 44% to be precise). Don't buy it.

2. Cholesterol. If it has some in it, that means it contains animal products. This one has 30 mg/serving. Don't buy this product.

3. Sodium. Rule of thumb, if the mg of sodium is less than the "Calories" per serving above, it's okay. This one is 470 mg per 250 calories/serving. Another reason not to buy it.

4. Dietary fiber. An essential nutrient, it plays a very important role in making your body work properly. We suggest that you look for products with lots of fiber. Another clue that this product contains animal-based foods is that it has zero fiber, which is contained ONLY in plant foods.

5. Sugars. We suggest you keep this to a minimum. It's almost impossible to buy packaged products like non-dairy milks or boxed cereal without lots of added sugar in them. This product has 5 grams of added sugar per serving. This is a product that you should not buy.

Ingredients List (for another product). In addition to the Nutrition Facts panel, this list will be somewhere on the package. Try to avoid packaged goods that have more than three or four ingredients. The list is ranked by weight of the ingredient. Here's one for a so-called "vegan cheese."

> INGREDIENTS: Soy Base (Filtered Water, Isolated Soy Protein), Casein* (A Dried Skim Milk Protein) Canola Oil, Modified Food Starch, Salt, Contains 2% or less of Rice Flour, Natural Flavors, Tapioca Starch, Sodium Polyphosphate, Powdered Cellulose, Tricalcium Phosphate, Sodium Phosphate, Mono and Diglycerides, Sorbic Acid (Preservative), Carrageenan, Sodium Citrate, Citric Acid, Lactic Acid, Vitamin A Palmitate, Vitamin C, Ferric Orthophosphate, Vitamin B12, Vitamin D3, Folic Acid, Vitamin B6, Riboflavin (Vitamin B2), Vitamin E, Potato Starch and Powdered Cellulose added to Prevent Caking. *Adds a trivial amount of Lactose.

This product actually has some animal products AND has far more than three ingredients—reinforcing the advice that "vegan meats and cheeses" should be minimized.

15

EATING OUTSIDE THE HOME

By J. Morris Hicks

Since most people consume half or more of their calories outside the home these days, it's very important that you learn how to eat "4Leaf style" while in restaurants, in social situations, in the workplace and while traveling.

Healthy Eating in Restaurants. You may be able to continue eating at your current favorite restaurants and just replace some of your usual entrées with other, more healthful, options on the menu. To be able to serve a healthy meal, however, a restaurant has to have fresh grains, vegetables, fruits and legumes in their kitchen.

Many restaurants, especially chain establishments, rely on meat, dairy and frozen foods for the majority of the meals they serve. The chef may have very little ability or willingness to adapt the menu. Not even Houdini could order a 4Leaf meal in one of those places! If one of those types of restaurants is a current favorite, you may need to find some new favorites that allow you to practice what we call "creative ordering."

Eight Simple Steps to 4Leaf Ordering

1. Look for any entrées that fit your new eating style. Some examples: teriyaki vegetables with brown rice, curried vegetables with chickpeas, or grilled eggplant on whole wheat pita bread. It is possible that there will be NO entrées that will work for you as is, but don't worry!

2. Check the menu entrées again, this time looking for a possible meal that would be great minus the meat and/or cheese. I call this the **"Tiger Shrimp, Hold the Shrimp"** technique. Years ago, I noticed an attractive dish on my yacht club menu called "Tiger Shrimp," served with whole grains, seaweed and a medley of garden-fresh vegetables. So, I simply told the waiter:

"I'll have the Tiger Shrimp, hold the shrimp, double up on the grains, vegetables and seaweed--AND kindly ask the chef to adjust the price accordingly."

The above anecdote illustrates how easy it can be to order 4Leaf meals in restaurants and save money at the same time. Listed at $22 on the menu, they charged me $12 every time.

As another example, I occasionally ask if the chef can substitute avocado for the bacon in the BLT. It now becomes an ALT. I make sure it is on whole wheat bread and that no mayonnaise is used. Not a great 4Leaf meal, but sometimes that's the best you can do in many casual dining establishments—like the snack bar at a large public park.

3. Look for healthy side dishes on the menu. Note: anything fried is *not* a healthy *side* since most of the calories will come from the oil! In addition to what you find in the "sides" portion of the menu, look at what veggies, grains,

potatoes and legumes accompany the various entrées. All of these are available in the kitchen and can be combined to make a fabulous meal.

4. Ask that your food be prepared with minimal or no oil.

5. Remember that the "token" vegetarian entrée is likely loaded with oil, white flour and cheese, derives very few calories from whole plants and is rarely close to being a even a 2Leaf or 3Leaf meal.

6. If you decide to order pasta, request that it be whole grain and that at least 2/3 of the dish is veggies. Also, verify that the sauce does not contain dairy or excessive oil, and consider asking for it to be served on the side. That way you won't eat as much of it.

7. If you are having bread with your meal, make sure that it is whole grain and that you don't use butter or olive oil.

8. Remember that a meal of vegetables (or fruit) without a grain, legume or potato will likely not have enough calories to keep you going for more than a few hours. Make sure you create a meal with "staying power."

After a little practice, this *creative ordering* can be a lot of fun.

And, regardless of what special meal you create, don't forget this magic, money-saving phrase: "Kindly ask the chef to adjust the price accordingly." Not only will you be enjoying healthy and delicious meals that you create yourself, you'll likely save money every time you dine. More on this in Chapter 17.

Healthy Eating in Social Situations

So what about parties and eating at friends' homes? This

can be more difficult but not impossible. Unless you know that there is going to be plenty of healthy food available, I strongly advise that you eat a healthy snack before you go.

If it's a cocktail party, simply dig into the carrots, broccoli, celery and hummus and avoid the cheese, shrimp and deviled eggs. Alternatively, you can always just enjoy a cocktail sans the solid food.

If it's a sit-down dinner, let your hosts know in advance that you are on a restricted diet. Politely stating that you don't want to inconvenience them in any way or have them adapt their menu for your needs helps to make this situation less awkward.

Depending on how well you know the host, you can offer to bring something to share that you know you can eat. Otherwise, eat enough before you go so that you are not very hungry.

Healthy Eating on the Road

While traveling, pack easy-to-eat items like apples, grapes, bananas, cherries or clementines. It is incredibly difficult to get a healthy meal at most rest stop fast food restaurants. At airports or shopping malls, look for the Mexican or Asian places. There you can usually get at least a 3Leaf meal, perhaps with a little more oil and salt than you would like. Sometimes, Subway might be your best bet—where you can get a veggie sandwich on whole wheat.

Another healthy option is the food buffet at many grocery chains like Whole Foods Market, Wegmans and many others. They always have a vast array of whole, plant-based foods that can either be eaten onsite or purchased to go. This method usually accounts for at least one of my meals each week.

Healthy Eating at the Workplace

Some combination of the following two ideas should work out for you:

1. Bring your own 4Leaf breakfast and/or lunch to work. Making it yourself is the best way to ensure you will have a healthy meal available. Want to eat your oatmeal at work? Place your oats in a container with raisins and almond milk or water. Then, cut up your fruit and put in another container. Mix them together when you are ready to eat. This works great whether eaten at your desk or in the cafeteria. You can warm it in the microwave at work or you can eat it cold like I do.

2. Check out your workplace cafeteria, where you hopefully can find some 4Leaf options for breakfast and/or lunch. You can use some of the above restaurant ordering techniques when telling the staff how you would like for them to make your sandwich.

When all else fails

We know that eating 4Leaf outside the home can sometimes be difficult and that occasionally you will simply not be able to find any suitable food at all. The good news is that, after you have been eating a near optimal diet for awhile, it will not be that painful to experience a little true hunger and just skip a meal from time to time. Just drink a little water and look forward to your next 4Leaf meal a few hours later.

Now, let's take a break and check up on how Tom Miller is doing.

16

PATIENT RETURNS ONE WEEK LATER

By Dr. Kerry Graff

KG: "So, what did you think about "Forks Over Knives?"

TM: "Wow, it makes a lot of sense. But it is hard to believe it is true when the government and doctors aren't talking about it. How come I haven't heard any of this before?"

KG: "I've been a doctor for twenty years and I just learned about all this in the last few years, although the data has been accumulating for decades. We are taught next to nothing about nutrition in medical school and residency. What we did learn was what the USDA recommends, but the USDA is really a farmer's advocacy group and doesn't base its recommendations primarily on health.

I bought into the same propaganda that you did--that "Milk does a body good" and that meat is a necessary source of protein. I had been encouraging patients, women especially, to get three servings of low fat milk products a day to help their bones. I was shocked to learn that people living in countries that eat the most dairy and meat have the WORST bones. I realized that I had been harming patients with my old advice. It is hard for doctors to open their minds to the idea that they have been wrong about something so important to health.

It also means that doctors have way less control over health than patients do, which is a blow to our egos, and also to our pocketbooks. We get paid for treating illness with pills and procedures, not for keeping people healthy in the first place by providing disease-preventing dietary advice. Let me assure you that the folks in the documentary aren't quacks and the science behind it is legitimate. How have you done with the diet changes I asked you to make?"

TM: "It wasn't that hard. I like oatmeal and soup anyway, so I was just swapping a tasty (but unhealthy) food that I enjoyed for a very healthy and even tastier one. I have a microwave at work, so it was easy to heat it up. My wife and I made a big pot of soup over the weekend. We also made veggie chili and had that for dinner on two of the nights. I had a few days when I didn't eat any meat, dairy or eggs at all! Cutting back on the alcohol has been a problem though. I really enjoy it."

KG: "What do you like so much about drinking wine?"

TM: "Well, I feel like I deserve it after a hard day at work. It helps me relax. My wife and I drink it together and we hang out, but she usually only drinks two glasses."

KG: "You do deserve to relax and to have an enjoyable time with your wife. What other ways do you relax and what other things do you enjoy doing together?"

TM: "I do yoga stretches on my own at home. It helps my back from the scoliosis. And my wife and I do a lot of bike riding and hiking together. I love that. Cooking together this past week, looking at recipes and menu planning has been fun, actually. We went online and found a bunch of whole food, plant-based recipes on the *Forks Over Knives* website to help us with dinner planning. I know you didn't ask me to move ahead with changing up dinners yet, but we got excited and just dove in. My energy is better. And all the vague stomach stuff I had been having is a lot better, too."

KG: "Great! Keep doing all that good stuff. You are lucky you have a partner on board with the diet changes you are making. It is really hard when a couple isn't doing this together. And yoga is terrific, both mentally and physically. Do you do the relaxation part of yoga as well as the stretches and does your wife do it with you?"

TM: "No. I don't and she doesn't. But she would probably love that. I'll ask her. Maybe we could do that for a half hour before we start making dinner together. I bet that would help me drink a little less wine."

KG: "Great idea! With the kidney stones, it is really important to stay well hydrated. Wine is a diuretic and actually dehydrates you. Maybe you could make sure to drink a large glass of water after yoga before you start drinking wine. And maybe you could limit it to one glass of wine before and one with dinner. If you are still feeling the need for some TLC (tender loving care) after your second glass of wine, you could try a hot cup of decaffeinated tea or coffee after the meal. Or maybe a little TLC from your wife. Sound doable?"

TM: "Oh yeah, I am willing to try that."

We redid the 4Leaf Survey and he was up to 18 (2Leaf level), likely getting between 40-60% of his calories from whole plant foods. Where did he still

need work? He was eating more whole grains, but a lot of them were processed like whole wheat bread and pasta. He was still using a lot of olive oil and drinking too much wine. There was still some meat and fish in his diet.

KG: "Tom, do you remember the Daily Reporting Version of the 4Leaf Survey in the back of the packet I gave you last week? Do you think you could score your points every day for the next month until your next visit, with a goal to get above 30 points every day? It will help you see what you are doing right and also where you are missing the mark.

Remember, you should count each glass of wine against your score as a sugar point. Your almond milk and the whole wheat bread or pastas you eat don't count against you, but also don't give you positive points. They may be plant-based, but they are processed, so not as healthy as whole foods. And you can sauté with any liquid. You don't need oil.

TM: "But isn't olive oil healthy?"

KG: "Well, it is healthier than some other oils but it is definitely NOT a health food. Remember the part in *Forks Over Knives* about endothelial cells in blood vessels? Any type of oil increases inflammation and makes plaque unstable. You already have plaque buildup in your arteries. You don't want more and you certainly don't want to make anything unstable and likely to rupture and form a clot."

TM: "Got it. Oil is out!"

KG: "You are making great progress, Tom. I can't wait to see how much more you have moved up the 4Leaf chart when I see you back in a month!"

17

$AVING MONEY WITH 4LEAF

By J. Morris Hicks

On the surface, it might appear that healthy eating will cost a lot more than our standard meat, dairy and egg diet. And since most people never get beneath the surface, the perceived high cost of plant-based eating just gives them one more reason not to give up their Typical Western Diet.

But for me, a 70-year old man enjoying vibrant health, I see things much differently. For a person who prepares his own food up until 6 p.m. and goes out to eat almost every night, I have actually saved money. Since I made the switch to plant-based eating in 2003, I calculate that I save around $400 per month--adding up to a total of almost $60,000 over the past 12 years. So how did I save that kind of money?

Two ways: by saving on the meals I prepare at home and saving even more money when I eat in restaurants. Let's begin with the typical meals that I prepare at home: my *Sailors Daily Oatmeal* and *Sailors Super Lunch or Dinner.* You can find both under "Recipes" at 4leafprogram.com.

It all boils down to cost per 100 calories. So, in preparation for this chapter, I visited my online grocer at PeaPod.com, where you can find the price, calories, percent fat, and fiber grams for every food that you can imagine. I then analyzed fourteen common foods, ranking them from least expensive to most expensive on a cost per 100 calories basis.

Notice in the chart below that by far, the least expensive foods are the grains and legumes. Since the bulk of my calories in both of my "go-to" meals are grains and legumes, averaging about 15 cents per 100 calories, it means that I can have a 500-calorie meal with over 300 of those 500 calories costing about 45 cents.

Even after adding a lot of the more expensive fruits and/or veggies (the other 200 calories), I can still prepare a pretty good meal (for one person) for around two or three dollars.

Food	$Cost per 100 calories	% Fat	Fiber
1. Brown Rice	.08	7%	A
2. Black Beans	.21	3%	A
3. Eggs	.28	57%	Zero
4. Cream Cheese	.30	80%	Zero
5. Wieners	.38	85%	Zero
6. Bacon	.38	75%	Zero
7. Chicken Breast	.55	17%	Zero
8. Apples	.62	3%	A
9. Cantaloupe	.69	5%	A
10. Oranges	.69	2%	A
11. Frozen Broccoli	.83	10%	A
12. Frozen Spinach	.93	10%	A
13. Fresh Broccoli	2.42	10%	A
14. Fresh Spinach	4.33	10%	A

What do we see here? Grains and legumes are great bargains. Averaging around 15 cents per 100 calories, low in fat and high in fiber, these are the kinds of foods that will keep you going between meals and won't break the bank.

What else do we see? The animal-based foods (3-7) are no bargain at any price. All are high in fat, loaded with cholesterol and have zero fiber or phytonutrients, all of which contribute to poor health.

What about those seemingly expensive vegetables at the bottom of the chart? Keep in mind that while you may put what seems like a lot of broccoli or spinach on your plate, they don't contain very many calories and will be a very small proportion of the total calories in the meal. They are loaded with health promoting vitamins, fiber and phytonutrients and you definitely should include them in your 4Leaf meals. Just don't let their cost per 100 calories scare you away!

Taking a look at fiber. Notice that all of the plant-based foods got an "A" in this category; whereas all five of the animal-based foods have absolutely no fiber. We need fiber, and we need much more than most of us are getting. The average American gets less than 10 grams of fiber daily, when experts recommend we get at least 25 grams per day. A whole food, plant-based diet will deliver more than 50 grams of fiber a day.

A word about starch. As Dr. McDougall says, "People have eaten a starch-based diet for thousands of years." They derived the bulk of their calories from grains, legumes and potatoes while eating as many fresh fruits and vegetables as they could find.

Without enough starch in our diet, we feel like we're

starving within a few hours after eating a plate of just fruits or just vegetables. Those starches also save us money.

Summary of savings with a plant-based diet. In the old days, I would eat a few sausage biscuits for breakfast and would grill some kind of meat when I had dinner at home. On a weekly basis, I would have about 12 meals at home and would eat 9 meals out. Believe it or not, it's those meals outside the home where I have saved the most money.

Savings at home. For my twelve weekly meals consumed at home, I computed an average cost of $3--compared to $5 per meal when I used to eat some combination of meat, dairy, eggs and/or fish at almost every home-cooked meal. With a savings of $2 per meal, I am now saving about $24 a week on those twelve meals.

Savings in restaurants. This is where I save the big bucks. In Chapter 15, I described my *creative ordering* process, where I order a $20 entrée, ask them to hold the meat, add a lot more of the grains and veggies, and to kindly adjust the price accordingly. By eating this way, I conservatively estimate that I save about $8 per meal. At nine meals a week, that works out to a $72 weekly savings.

Summary of Annual Savings

- $1248 saved at home. (52x24=1248)
- $3744 saved eating out. (52x72=3744)
- $4992 Annual Savings

What could you do with an extra five grand a year? Install solar panels on your roof, take a great vacation, put aside money for retirement or your kids' college education, or give to your favorite charity?

The Hidden Costs of Animal Foods. In addition to that five grand per year, you will also save money on medical bills, prescription drugs, vitamins, lost work and income due to illness and so much more. If you add up all the factors involved, eating a whole food, plant-based diet is one of the best bargains that you will experience in your lifetime. Then, when you consider the many benefits of "vibrant health" for yourself while doing great things for the environment, there is simply no comparison.

Avoid cans and save even more money. Not only do those containers almost double the cost of the contents, they're also an environmental nightmare. I did a little analysis of canned vs. dried beans. Here's what I found:

> The canned beans cost $.35 per 100 calories compared to only $.21 for the dried beans. If I eat 100 calories of beans every day, each year I save $51.10 by using the dry beans that come in a bag.

What about the environmental impact? In the USA alone, we use 37 billion cans each year. If we didn't use cans at all, we could save enough energy to power 36 million homes. We'd also save an enormous amount of water and finite metal materials. That said, the impact of eating animal-based foods is monumental compared to eating plant-based even with using cans. So if you just can't manage to soak and cook your own beans (my co-author is guilty here), then use cans and recycle.

Want to see the full analysis on hpjmh.com? Just Google "Canned or Dried Morris Hicks." In fact, if you want to find what I have written on almost any topic, just include the two words "Morris Hicks" in your query. One or more of my 900+ blog-posts will probably appear.

18

WHAT ABOUT PROTEIN?

By J. Morris Hicks

If you're like most people, you may have been wondering about that question since you started reading this book. And, if you decide to adopt the 4Leaf lifestyle, this is the question you will likely hear every single day for the rest of your life:

"Where do you get your protein?"

You will hear this question from family, friends, co-workers, doctors and occasionally from complete strangers. Please don't answer flippantly, as many who ask you the question will actually have genuine concerns about your health if you don't get enough protein. So you want to give them a serious response.

Suggested responses to that very common question:

"From the same place that some of the strongest animals in the world (elephants, giraffes, horses, hippos, etc.) get theirs. From whole plants."

"Actually, plants have a lot more protein than most people think. Did you know that broccoli is 40% protein and that calorie for calorie, spinach has more protein than sirloin?"

"Like the gorilla, our closest relative in the wild, I get my protein from whole plants."

"Even vegetables containing the least protein have more than enough for humans. It's virtually impossible not to get enough protein as long as you are eating sufficient calories."

"Many cultures throughout the world live their entire lives eating little, if any, animal products—they are not only strong, their incidence of chronic illnesses like cancer and heart disease is near zero."

To summarize, we have many things to worry about in life, but getting enough protein in our diet is not one of them.

So why is everyone so worried about getting enough protein? Because of the long history of advertising by the meat, dairy, egg and fish industries. All of their products contain only two macronutrients (fat and protein) and it surely wouldn't be good marketing to promote the first one.

What is the optimal amount of protein in our diets? The Recommended Daily Allowance, RDA (note this is *recommended* amount and not a *minimum* amount) is 0.8 mg protein/kilogram, which translates to about 8-10% of our calories. This RDA was based on data showing that virtually every individual functions well on 8-10% dietary protein and that protein intake over 10% is associated with increased incidence of many chronic diseases.

So protein consumption over 10% is actually *bad* for me? Yes. It is associated with significant increased risk of cancer, heart disease, kidney disease and autoimmune disorders. I should clarify that it is virtually impossible to get too much protein if you're getting it ONLY from plant-based sources. And even if you do, it doesn't cause the problems that are associated with too much animal protein.

But won't eating more protein make me stronger and faster? No. Numerous studies have shown that athletes actually do better when they switch from a high protein diet to a plant-based one that is 10% protein. Many pro athletes have taken these studies to heart and are now cleaning up the court, so to speak. Just ask Serena Williams.

If you need more reassurance that a plant-based diet won't make you weak and puny, check out Mac Danzig, Brendan Brazier, Patrik Bobaumain, Scott Jurek and Rich Roll.

Can't I get my 10% protein from animal sources? No. Animal-based foods are all much higher in protein than 10%. There is no way to eat animal foods without getting a higher than recommended amount of protein in your diet.

For more "protein" information, see Chapter 29.

19

OMEGA-3, CALCIUM, IRON, VITAMIN D AND B12

By Dr. Kerry Graff

In addition to protein, there are a few other nutrients that people are concerned about when they consider adopting a plant-based diet. In this chapter, I draw on the collective wisdom of Dr. T. Colin Campbell and the five medical doctors featured in the first three chapters of "Healthy Eating, Healthy World"--Drs. Caldwell Esselstyn, John McDougall, Dean Ornish, Neal Barnard, and Joel Fuhrman.

The good news is that you don't ever need to eat ANY animal-based foods in order to get all the vitamins and minerals you need. And you probably won't need much supplementation either, with the exception of B12 and possibly Vitamin D.

Here are five frequently asked questions that I hear in my office along with my replies:

1. Don't I need omega-3 fatty acids from fish or fish oil supplements? This was addressed when going over the survey. Basically, you get a perfect ratio of omega-3 to omega-6 from eating whole plants and do not need to do anything specific to be sure you obtain extra omega-3. In addition, a recent meta-analysis showed no survival benefit from taking fish oil supplements, despite the billion dollars or more per year that we spend on them.

Another recent study showed many fish oil supplements are contaminated with heavy metals, which are toxic. Just throw them out and never buy them again! If you remain concerned about getting enough omega-3 while eating a plant-based diet, some good plant-based sources of this nutrient are walnuts and flax, chia, and hemp seeds, but you *do not need them.*

2. Don't I need calcium from dairy to prevent osteoporosis? Thanks to an enormous amount of advertising by the dairy industry, just about everyone believes eating dairy builds strong bones. In reality, nothing could be further from the truth. In fact, countries with the highest dairy consumption have the highest rates of osteoporosis and bone fractures! How can this be?

The consumption of animal protein (in the form of animal flesh as well as calcium-rich dairy products) actually promotes bone loss. Proteins from plants do not have this blood acidifying effect. Our bodies can't tolerate this and pull calcium out of our bones to neutralize the acid (think Tums). Plant proteins have different properties than animal proteins and don't cause the blood acidity. Thus, they do not contribute to bone loss.

The experts mentioned above agree that minimizing calcium loss by avoiding animal-based foods is far more important for bone health than maximizing calcium intake. By eating a diet of whole plants, it would be impossible for you not to get enough calcium (as well as all of the other minerals you require) as long as you avoid the animal products that deplete the calcium from your bones.

3. Don't I need to drink milk to get Vitamin D?
Vitamin D occurs naturally in very few foods and milk is
not one of them. However, cow's milk, like many soy and
nut milks, is fortified with Vitamin D and the dairy
industry has been doing that for so long, that people
naturally assume that they need to drink cow's milk to get
enough Vitamin D.

Technically, Vitamin D is not a vitamin, but a hormone
produced by sunlight on your skin. That is the way nature
intended humans to acquire Vitamin D and, if possible, is
the way we should get it. When Vitamin D is made in the
skin, there is a mechanism that prevents us from
accumulating too much, even if we get a lot of sun
exposure. Taking supplements of Vitamin D in the form
of pills bypasses the system that prevents excessive storage
and levels can become toxic.

Living in upstate New York, however, many of my
patients aren't going to be making Vitamin D in their skin
much of the year. In addition to having a lot of cloudy
days, we often work jobs that keep us inside. We cover up
to stay warm and, even if we do go outside when the
weather is warm enough to show some skin, many of us
slather ourselves with sunscreen. While this may keep our
skin from frying, it also blocks all the Vitamin D
formation! So, should I encourage my patients to take a
supplement, at least in the winter months, to keep their
levels in a "normal range?"

Well, let's see what the experts say. The US Preventive
Services Task Force, an independent organization that
evaluates the effectiveness of various treatments,
concluded that there is insufficient evidence to conclude
for or against taking Vitamin D as a supplement--unless

you are over 65 and at increased risk of falls, in which case they recommend it.

Until we have more specific data, I will be happy to write everyone a prescription to go to Florida for at least a week in the winter to stock up on their Vitamin D! Joking aside, get some sun on skin that hasn't been covered with sunscreen--enough to get a little color but not enough to burn--whenever you can. That rule works well, since light-skinned people need less sun to generate their Vitamin D than darker skinned people and UV penetration depends on time of the year and time of day, along with other factors.

4. Don't I need to eat meat to prevent anemia? Once again, a varied diet rich in whole, plant-based foods will provide you with all the iron that you need to make red blood cells. Although red meat does contain a lot of iron, it also has a lot of fat, cholesterol and animal protein (which you now know is *not* a good thing) which don't tag along when you are getting iron from plant sources. In addition, iron overload is a significant problem in people eating SAD, causing additional health problems. With plants, you get enough iron but not too much.

5. Aren't plant-based diets deficient in Vitamin B12? This is where you might want to take a routine supplement or at least monitor the levels in your blood occasionally. Vitamin B12 is actually made by the bacteria in dirt. Why didn't nature put this vital nutrient in plants? She did in that she didn't plan on our food consumption to take place in such a sterile environment!

Our ancestors weren't so meticulous about washing their vegetables and got B12 from dirt or insects in some of their foods. We do not recommend you eat bugs or dirt!!!

Please wash those fruits and veggies well, especially if you buy non-organic ones that have been treated with pesticides!

If you had been eating meat until you read this book, you likely have several years of B12 in storage. That is because animal-based foods contain Vitamin B12 because animals eat dirty plants. After a couple of years of eating a whole food, plant-based diet, you may need to start replacing B12.

That said, many plant-based foods are now fortified with B12 (almond milk, for example) so you may not need to take it in a pill at all, depending on how much of these B12 fortified foods you eat. Your doctor can check your level and let you know how much, if any, you need. 400mcg daily is usually enough and you may not even need that much.

The Bottom Line. You will get nearly everything your body needs from a whole food, plant-based diet. Other than a B12 supplement and possibly Vitamin D depending on your circumstances, in my opinion, practically all other vitamin supplements are a complete waste of money and are even potentially harmful! Taken as supplements, vitamins are not in the same combinations and proportions as they are found in nature.

For example, foods that contain a lot of beta-carotene decrease risk of cancer, but beta-carotene supplements on their own were shown to actually increase the risk for cancer! Just another reminder not to fool with Mother Nature.

20

IT'S TIME TO TALK WITH YOUR DOCTOR

By J. Morris Hicks

Before you begin to make big changes in the way you are eating, there is one more topic that we need to cover-- talking with your medical doctor. Perhaps you've already seen this message on the copyright page:

> **CAUTION**. Eating the 4Leaf way (described throughout this book) may quickly decrease your need for medications. You should tell your physician what you're doing. If he/she is not familiar with, or skeptical of, this eating style, please direct him or her to plantrician.org or nutritionstudies.org.

Why is it so important to involve your physician? Because it is imperative that appropriate adjustments are made to any medications that you might be taking, because you are likely to need far less of them rather quickly. This is particularly true for diabetes and high blood pressure medications. You will see an example of this in the next chapter.

When you first mention to your physician that you are in

the process of adopting a whole food, plant-based diet, you are far more likely to hear words of caution than encouragement. There are two primary reasons behind that likely response:

1. It's not how most doctors eat. In all likelihood, your doctor and his/her family eat some combination of meat, dairy, eggs and fish on a routine basis and, like almost everyone else, they truly believe that they need to eat some animal protein to be healthy. That's because of the "protein myth" that we cover in Chapter 29.

2. It's not what they're taught. Despite a mountain of scientific and clinical evidence that a whole food, plant-based diet supports optimal health, it is not yet part of the curriculum in our schools of medicine. But that hasn't prevented a host of pioneering doctors from guiding their patients through the process of taking charge of their own health--just by changing what they eat. You can take charge of your own health too.

If your physician is discouraging you from adopting a whole food, plant-based diet, ask him or her if he/she is familiar with the works of Caldwell Esselstyn, MD (Cleveland Clinic), Dean Ornish, MD (UCSF) and T. Colin Campbell, PhD (Cornell). They are the three experts (medical and scientific) who influenced President Clinton to adopt a similar diet, saying he did so "to reverse his heart disease" in 2010.

If your doctor is knowledgeable about this way of eating and can give you a valid reason why you should not adopt this diet (such as you have diverticulitis) please listen and heed. If not, please don't let your doctor deter you from adopting the diet eaten by the healthiest people on Earth.

If your doctor is not familiar with the health benefits of a whole food, plant-based diet, please encourage him/her to check out the work of the doctors listed above and perhaps watch *Forks Over Knives*. For more information, he/she can review the information at plantrician.org and nutritionstudies.org.

In their defense. Doctors make up one of the most highly respected groups of professionals in the world. Most of them enter the medical field to help people, and they spend many years and lots of money educating themselves for a career in their chosen field. Later, they find themselves trapped in a system that promotes profits over health and confusion over clarity.

In reality, the United States currently has a "Disease Care System" rather than a "Health Care System." This system trains and pays physicians to do tests, conduct procedures and prescribe drugs once disease has struck and it provides little training in, or reimbursement for, keeping people healthy in the first place. Philosopher Wendell Berry describes how our medical system treats the topic of food:

People are fed by the food industry, which pays no attention to health--and are treated by the health industry, which pays no attention to food.

In the future, physicians' incomes will be tied directly to the health of their patients and then they WILL be "paying attention to food." But why wait when you have the opportunity to change your health for the better today?

You might want to mention to your doctor that it would be great to have a physician who understands the role of nutrition in health and is helping patients take steps to prevent or reverse up to 80% of the chronic diseases they might encounter in their lifetime.

On your next visit, ask your doctor if he or she has taken the time to read any of the works of Esselstyn, Ornish or Campbell or to watch *Forks Over Knives*. You might also want to leave him/her a copy of Dr. Graff's letter to all of her fellow medical providers in Chapter 37.

Finally, are you thinking about getting a new doctor who truly "gets it" about food? For a registry of medical practitioners who are dedicated to integrating plant-based nutrition into their practices, visit plantbaseddocs.com for a searchable directory.

21

TYPE 2 DIABETES SUCCESS STORY

By Dr. Kerry Graff

Mrs. Bentley weighed nearly 300 pounds and was at her wit's end. I sent her to an endocrinologist for her diabetes several years prior because her sugars were so difficult to control, but she returned to my office that day completely discouraged. Here's how she greeted me:

> "My sugars are high, so the endocrinologist increases my insulin. My sugars get better for a few weeks, but then go up again and I have to increase the insulin even more. I'm on over 100 units and four shots a day now! And the insulin causes me to gain more and more weight! The endocrinologist says this is just what happens with diabetes. I hate it!"

In addition to diabetes, she suffered from high blood pressure, heart disease, reflux, degenerative joint disease and neuropathy, which caused a painful burning sensation in her legs. Her medical conditions severely impacted her quality of life. I told her that I recently learned how effective a low fat, whole food, plant-based diet is in treating diabetes and asked her if she wanted to give it a try. At that point, I think she would have tried just about anything.

I had her take the 4Leaf Survey, and despite the fact that she was following the American Diabetic Association (ADA) diet, she scored only at the *Better Than Most* level. We mapped out a plan for the diet changes I was asking her to make. "But I'll be eating a lot of carbs! Isn't that going to make my diabetes worse?" she asked.

KG: "It is counterintuitive, for sure. All these years you have been told to avoid them, and now I'm telling you that you should be eating **mostly** carbs! But this type of diet was shown by Dr. Neal Barnard to reduce sugars three times better than the ADA diet you have been on.

First of all, carbs are not all the same. Good carbohydrates are ones that are as close to the way they come in nature as possible. Our bodies know what to do with those kinds of carbs.

It is the processed carbs—the crackers, white bread, pastries, cakes and candies--that our bodies have no idea how to handle and cause our shoot blood sugars to shoot up. Basically, focus on eating carbs that only have one ingredient on the label. Or better yet, carbs that don't even need a label!"

In addition, fat in your diet increases insulin resistance. Insulin works like a key to open the door for sugar to get into cells. Fat gums up the lock, making it hard for insulin to do its job. Reducing fat in your diet will help insulin work better."

Before she left the office, I reminded her that the diet changes she was going to make would likely reduce her need for medication (especially for insulin) quickly and significantly. As such, I told her that she should let her endocrinologist know what she was doing, cut back on insulin per her instructions and continue to check her sugars four times a day, plus anytime she had symptoms. She was due back in a month but was to call or see me sooner for any problems or questions.

Mrs. Bentley was a quick learner and highly motivated. She went right to eating at the 3 to 4Leaf level. Within a week, she called to tell me her systolic blood pressure, which had been 140 when I saw her, had dropped to 90 and she was dizzy. We decreased one of her three blood pressure meds. At her follow-up appointment one month later, she was positively gleeful.

"I feel great! I have so much energy! "

The increased fiber (basically she had increased this 500% by eating 4Leaf) had caused some mild gas and bloating initially, but that had all resolved. She definitely didn't need medication for constipation anymore! She wasn't dizzy, but on exam, her systolic blood pressure was still low, so we reduced her blood pressure medication further. Then I asked her about her sugars:

"I am off over half my insulin already! I can't believe it. I feel better than I have in years. I have my life back! Just by changing what I eat!"

After years of feeling like a victim of disease, she was now feeling empowered. Patients have way more control over their health by what they put on their forks than doctors do with the pills and procedures they prescribe. I think that is the biggest realization for all of us.

Mrs. Bentley's story continues. She, like all of us, is a work in progress. As she continues this way of eating, she needs less medication and her weight comes down. Her joints hurt less. She is able to be more active. Each positive step results in further health improvements. She is no longer on the downward spiral of disease but rather on the upward spiral of regaining her health.

Mrs. Bentley changed the story of her life by adopting a whole food, plant-based diet. You can too!

My thoughts about the ADA Diet. Mentioned earlier, that's the one recommended by the American Diabetes Association for "managing your disease." Here's why I don't think that diet is such a good idea.

Let's begin with the three macronutrient sources for calories: carbohydrates, fats and protein. When you eat less from one source, you need to eat a higher percentage of the others to get adequate calories to fuel your body. In the ADA diet, where carbohydrates are highly restricted to control blood sugars, a large percentage of the calories come from fat and protein.

Is it any wonder that most diabetics don't die from uncontrolled sugars but rather from heart disease (related to the fat they ingest) and kidney disease (related to their animal protein intake)? Honestly, what good is sugar control to a diabetic if they have a heart attack or their kidneys fail?

The good news is that 4Leaf eating is good for almost everything--except for keeping your doctor in business!

22

GLUTEN-FREE ON 4LEAF?

By Dr. Kerry Graff

The 4Leaf way of eating is great for almost all of our chronic diseases: heart disease, diabetes, autoimmune disorders, kidney disease, and cancer--without needing modification. Gluten intolerance is an exception.

Gluten is a protein found in wheat and related grains like rye and barley. Most people have no problem eating gluten-containing foods and they are a good source of nutrients and calories. But some people will develop diarrhea, abdominal pain and other issues if they eat gluten. The most serious form of this is Celiac Disease, a genetic condition in which the body makes antibodies against gluten that then attack the lining of the intestine. Obviously, this is a pretty serious disorder! If you have been diagnosed with Celiac Disease through blood tests or biopsy, avoid gluten at all costs!

SAD contains a lot of gluten, primarily in the processed foods that we eat. Many people who eat SAD feel significantly better when they go gluten-free and thus assume they must be gluten intolerant. However, processed foods contain a lot of substances in addition to gluten (sugar substitutes, preservatives, dyes, etc.) that can cause GI unhappiness. Many people improve, not because they are avoiding gluten, but because they are not ingesting other things in processed foods. These folks will do great on a whole food, plant-based diet that is not gluten-free.

Some people, however, truly do have gluten intolerance and need to avoid it. The good news is that you can still eat 4Leaf and get all of its wonderful health benefits even if you really must also be gluten-free. You will just need to avoid the foods you know you shouldn't eat. Because gluten is so pervasive in packaged foods, I highly recommend anyone who is diagnosed with gluten intolerance to see a qualified nutritionist to learn how to detect and avoid it. Be sure to let him or her know that in addition to going gluten-free, you also want to go meat, dairy and egg-free!

So, what's the best approach for someone eating SAD and having gut problems? Abdominal complaints in folks eating SAD are incredibly common and testing all of these folks for Celiac Disease would be extremely expensive. My recommendation is that if your abdominal symptoms are severe with chronic diarrhea or weight loss, see your doctor and get tested to rule out celiac and other serious diseases now, before embarking on your 4Leaf transition.

If your gut symptoms are milder, I would recommend that you transition to the 4Leaf diet without avoiding glutens and see if your symptoms resolve. The vast majority of the time they will. If you continue to have symptoms, see your doctor before going gluten-free, as the antibody test that confirms celiac disease decreases the longer you avoid gluten. This means that if you have been gluten-free for several months, you may test negative for celiac disease even if you actually have it.

23

EVIDENCE OF DETOX

By J. Morris Hicks

As vibrant health begins to permeate your body, you may very well witness some evidence of detox along the way. I did, and I wasn't expecting it.

After eating the Standard American Diet for 58 years, I switched to the 4Leaf level of a whole food, plant-based diet in a matter of weeks. Since the *natural* detoxification that I experienced was unexpected, my goal here is to help you be prepared for, and indeed welcome, the natural process of your body healing itself.

One of the first changes you will notice is that you will no longer need any reading material in the bathroom. While on that topic, you may also notice some colors, textures and odors that you've never experienced before. This is just nature doing her work.

In early 2003, in addition to making radical changes in my diet, I also looked into the possibility of having a colonic hydrotherapy treatment. If you're not familiar with the procedure, they basically put a tube in your rear end and clean out your entire colon with a whole lot of water. Also referred to as a colonic irrigation, I was told that lots of movie stars have the procedure on a regular basis as it helps with their appearance. So I scheduled a treatment but later canceled it.

Why? Because I noticed that my body was taking care of that cleansing process all by itself. Now that I was feeding it lots of fiber and phytonutrients at every meal (instead of a steady intake of toxins), my body began the process of cleaning house.

And I began to notice the evidence of that process in my stool--seeing stuff that I had never seen before. Noticing that Mother Nature was taking care of business herself convinced me to cancel my colonic appointment and never reschedule it.

Nature at work. Think about the incredibly complex task that nature conducts continuously--the task of replacing practically ALL of the 100 trillion cells in your body every ten years. In going about her work of nurturing and replacing cells, nature manages a nonstop detoxification program of her own--IF you give her the right food.

Emergence of vibrant health. After detoxifying your body, you will likely notice other signs of vibrant health emerging:

- Clearer complexion. Even at age 58, I was still plagued with a fairly minor case of acne on a regular basis. Then, all of a sudden, it disappeared. I had blamed it on my oily skin, when in reality, it was the toxins in every pore of my body.
- Better facial color. Instead of looking old and gray, your skin will start having a youthful glow.
- Sometimes hair color and eyesight improves as well!
- Weight loss. Almost everyone experiences weight loss

if they are carrying extra weight. More on that in the next chapter.

- Improved sleep and better energy.
- Less bad breath and body odor.
- You will be sick a lot less frequently. When you do come down with an illness, it will likely be much milder and you will probably recover much more quickly. All of those fruits and vegetables provide phytonutrients that fight off disease!

You see, all of the above conditions primarily result from a toxin-loaded diet and will probably disappear when you let nature start keeping those 100 trillion cells healthy and clean.

So when you begin noticing evidence of detox, don't be alarmed! Soon you are going to see first-hand the miracle of vibrant health starting in your body. It's almost like giving your automobile the kind of fuel recommended by the manufacturer--for the very first time.

Speaking of cars, consider that most people give much more thought to the type of fuel that they put in their vehicles than to the fuel that they put in their bodies. Can you imagine how your new BMW would run if you put a mixture of kerosene, milk and Gatorade in its tank? Sound absurd? It's no more absurd than us humans getting only 7% of our calories from whole plants, when nature designed us to get 80% or more from those foods.

Making every bite count. Back in 2005, I decided to count all of my bites for a few days and then ran the numbers. Based on the roughly ten trillion cells that my body replaces each year, I computed that the future health of 100 million cells was riding on every single bite I put in my mouth.

I now try to think about my "bite-counting exercise" when making a decision whether or not to chow down on some junk food.

A final bonus. There's one more piece of evidence that I would like to present before wrapping up this chapter. As nature goes about cleaning out all of the cells along your thousands of miles of arteries, she touches every single part of the body. And blood flow improves everywhere, not just in your coronary arteries. For men, this means that you and your partner might soon be in for a little more action in the bedroom.

The Bottom Line. If you get serious about what you put in your mouth, Mother Nature will get serious about rewarding you with vibrant health. And that will probably include some effortless and permanent weight-loss that we will cover in the next chapter.

24

LOSING WEIGHT WITH 4LEAF

By J. Morris Hicks

First of all, 4Leaf is not a weight-loss diet. It is an eating concept based on the pursuit of vibrant health--for ourselves and for our planet. Conveniently, if your goal is vibrant health, one of the many benefits of eating high on the 4Leaf scale is effortless and permanent weight-loss.

You feed your body what it needs for vibrant health and it will automatically seek its ideal weight. So why are there so many overweight vegetarians? Because many of them eat a lot more processed foods and a lot fewer whole plants than you might think--at least until they take the 4Leaf Survey!

Although some don't admit it, the vast majority of folks make changes in their diet for one primary reason--to lose weight. Even those who truly make the changes in the pursuit of vibrant health, are a little disappointed if they don't see the weight-loss they were expecting.

This chapter was designed to help people maximize their chances of enjoying the ideal weight and body that they are seeking. It all boils down to just four things: breakfast, lunch, dinner and snacks! Being creatures of habit, it's time to start forming some healthy new eating habits for all of your routine meals and snacks. Let's take a look at each one and start thinking about how you're going to put more whole plants in all of those meals that you eat regularly.

Breakfast. As the most important meal of the day, it's really critical to make sure that your *routine* breakfast derives well over 80% of its calories from whole plants. An aspiring 4Leaf friend of mine hasn't been able to lose all of her excess weight, and she typically begins her day with a toasted English muffin and peanut butter. **Red flag #1.**

For starters, the English muffin is not a whole plant and at best, even the "low fat" peanut butter is over 55% fat; regular is over 70%. That combination has no chance of promoting weight-loss. We recommend that you get real serious about this extremely important meal and make those first few bites of the day among your healthiest.

Lunch and Dinner. For some people, lunch is the big meal of the day and for others, it's dinner. Whatever it is for you, we once again recommend that you take the time to make sure that your *routine* meals (things you eat several times a week) are mostly whole plants with less than 20% fat. Here are a few things to consider when eating at lunch or dinner at home or in restaurants:

1. Make sure that your salad is not mostly fat. Most of the calories in restaurant salads do not come from whole plants. They come from the dressing and the ubiquitous cheese. Even 100% plant-based salads usually derive over half their calories from the salad dressing or olive oil. And if you eliminate that dressing, your salad likely won't have enough calories to last you for two hours. So just add some grains, legumes or potatoes and you'll be fine.

2. Pasta is rarely a 4Leaf meal. We find that aspiring 4Leaf-ers who load up on pasta and bread at every meal have trouble achieving the weight-loss they might be expecting. The problem is that neither pasta nor bread is a whole plant, in nature's package. That doesn't mean you can't eat pasta and bread, but you will need to do a little tweaking to make it a healthy meal.

When ordering pasta, we suggest telling the waiter that you would like to have a small "side" of whole grain pasta without the cream sauce. Then ask for a full-size plate of vegetables along with a small portion of whole grain bread. While this meal may be only in the 3Leaf range (70% of calories from whole plants), the "menu version" of pasta primavera will typically not even score at the 1Leaf level. Remember my aspiring 4Leaf friend? She continues to eat lots of pasta (usually not even whole wheat) and is still not adding many vegetables. **Red Flag #2.**

3. Think whole veggies, grains and legumes when you think about lunch or dinner. And get into a habit of really loading up on the veggies. Then, since those veggies have very few calories, just add some of the starchy foods to prevent getting hungry between meals.

4. Go easy on the non 4Leaf snacks. Many people get a greater percentage of their calories than they would care to admit--munching on snacks between meals. If you want to lose weight, most of those snacks must be at the 4leaf level. As for my aspiring 4Leaf friend, still remaining in her home is a vast array of cookies, salty snacks, nuts, and all manner of sweets. **Red Flag #3.**

Remember the shopping rule: "If it goes in your shopping cart, it will end up in your stomach." In her case, I suggested developing a few healthy 4Leaf snacks that she would truly enjoy. Maybe home-made hummus with carrots and celery for dipping. Why home-made? Because it's darn near impossible to find packaged hummus in the grocery store that's not loaded with fat from the added oil.

It all begins with discipline; then, when the new healthy eating habits take over, you'll be well on your way to vibrant health--and the trim body you're seeking. (See Appendix C, D, E and F for more ideas.)

Quick story. My son Jason does some moonlighting as a personal trainer and health coach. One of his long-term clients was a doctor (5' 8") who was a bit overweight at 210 pounds. After three years of routine workouts in the gym, and minimal weight-loss, Brian said that he was ready to try that "4Leaf thing" that Jason had told him about.

So, in addition to the routine workouts, they began a 60-day regimen of Brian reporting what he ate each day on an Excel spreadsheet. Jason analyzed and scored all the food and reported back to Brian his daily 4Leaf level via email--with this reminder at the bottom of each message:

"It's not about weight-loss, it's all about vibrant health. The weight-loss will take care of itself."

Six months later, Brian weighed 160 pounds, after not EVER being under 185 since he was 13. As he went below 180, people kept asking him what his weight goal was. He kept telling them, "My goal is vibrant health, the weight is taking care of itself." The vibrant health also enabled him to eliminate all of his meds, including one for gout.

Several years later, Brian is still enjoying vibrant health and a trim body. He even announced to his entire staff in public (with us there) that Jason Hicks had saved his life.

Need more help? Dr. Graff offers a few more tips:

1. Be honest with yourself about what you're really eating.
2. It's tough to eat 4Leaf (and lose weight) if you still have oil in your diet. It packs 100 calories of fat per tablespoon. It's almost ubiquitous these days: hummus, salad dressing, vegan mayo, etc. Get it out of your diet.
3. Get serious about limiting the heavily processed "whole grain" products in your diet: crackers, bread, pasta, etc.
4. Make water your go-to drink. Most other drinks (juices, plant-milks, alcohol) have lots of calories and no fiber.
5. Even smoothies, which may be 100% whole plants, can cause your body to consume too many calories before feeling full. Drinking these slowly can offset that issue.
6. Although they are whole plants, avocados, olives, nuts and seeds are all very high in fat content and loaded with calories. Limit these if you want to lose weight.
7. Get serious about exercise. See Chapter 35.
8. If you are doing all of the above and are still not progressing to your ideal weight, see your physician. Certain medical conditions or medications may be the problem.

The Bottom Line. Having trouble losing the weight you expected? As with Brian, it's mainly about the food. And it typically boils down to not enough whole fruits, vegetables, grains and legumes and way too much white pasta, olive oil, bread, salty snacks, French fries, onion rings, sweets, alcohol and high fat whole plants like nuts, seeds, olives and avocados.

Get serious about all of these things and you are likely to be rewarded with the trim body that you're seeking.

25

WHY DO I CRAVE UNHEALTHY FOODS?

By Dr. Kerry Graff

Are you craving fatty or sweet foods? Don't beat yourself up! You are just being human. For almost all of the 200,000 years of human existence, eating calorically dense sweet and fatty foods was actually a healthy and necessary thing to do.

Eating these foods when they were available (which was rare) and storing them as fat helped our ancestors survive during the times when food was not plentiful. Those who didn't have such a strong drive to eat these foods were less likely to live long enough to reproduce. So this "craving" for sweet and fatty foods is hardwired into our DNA.

Our environment has changed, however. Instead of sweet and fatty foods being a rare find as in our ancestors' day, they are now EVERYWHERE--and often they are even cheap to boot! And, at least in the western world, few people experience periods of famine.

Hopefully, this information will help you see how this biologic trait that helped us survive in the past is now killing us, by making us obese and riddling us with chronic disease! The bad news is that you aren't going to be able to change thousands of years of genetic selection. The good news is that humans have a cerebral cortex, which means we are smart enough to figure out why we do what we do and to CHOOSE differently.

In addition, most people who adopt a 4Leaf diet feel great very quickly. This is positive reinforcement for doing the right things that bring them good health. When they fall off the wagon and eat things they crave, they often feel really lousy (physically and mentally) afterwards. And that is negative reinforcement to help us resist those cravings.

Finally, as more people realize what is happening, we will hopefully change our environment as well. Instead of golden arches on every corner, we may find 4Leaf Cafes. I'd love to see that day!

26

SPOUSES, CHILDREN AND ROOMMATES

By J. Morris Hicks

Without a doubt, the single biggest obstacle to fully embracing the whole food, plant-based 4Leaf lifestyle is an unsupportive spouse or significant other. And that is why Dr. Caldwell Esselstyn will not accept new heart-disease reversal patients in his program unless their spouses accompany them to the initial training and orientation sessions at the Wellness Institute of The Cleveland Clinic.

Does this mean that you should drop the whole idea if your spouse is not on board? No, but it's going to take more time. You'll need that time to do everything within your power to help him/her understand why you are so excited about embracing this revolutionary way of eating. Regardless of how much time it takes, it will be well worth it. After all, what could be more important than vibrant health for both of you?

Can you make the change on your own? Yes, but it's much easier for a single person to do this than it is for someone who is married to an unsupportive spouse. That's because when you make a change in the way you are eating, you are affecting a significant portion of the waking hours you spend together. And that is a VERY big deal. Also, your spouse may very well be the person who does all the shopping and/or the cooking.

To be sure, this new adventure will be much more rewarding if you are both on the same page. Hence, you should do all that you can to start this life-changing journey together. As you share reading material and gently urge your spouse to join you, you should always be respectful as you appeal for his/her priceless support.

At the end of the day, a delicately balanced combination of listening, supporting, loving, understanding and caring will probably be the most convincing. As I said, this process may take some time so just be prepared to be patient. The stakes are high and they deserve your very best efforts.

What about the children? Teaching them a powerful, health-promoting way of eating while they are young is undoubtedly the best lifetime gift that you could possibly give them. It basically means that you're empowering them and all those who follow--with the ability to avoid chronic disease and live a long, healthy and happy life. But it won't be easy with barriers like these on the typical kids menu:

Menu Item	Fat %	Cholesterol	Fiber
Cheeseburger	32%	40 mg	1g
Cheese Pizza	43%	10 mg	1g
Chicken Nuggets	53%	34 mg	0
Mac & Cheese	40%	10 mg	1g

The good news is that it's not that difficult to change their habits if they're five or under. Unfortunately, your task will become increasingly more difficult as they grow older. It's also much easier if you don't have to share the children with unsupportive ex-spouses.

Consider cutting yourself some slack. Everyone loves their children and wants the best for them, yet there are times when we are just unable to get them to embrace a health-promoting diet, despite our best efforts. If the barriers are just too many and too high when it comes to your kids, Kerry and I recommend that you not be too hard on yourself.

While your kids may not choose to embrace your new diet-style as soon as you would like, there's no need to add unnecessary stress to your own lives by trying to force the issue too soon. Just model the behavior that you would like for them to adopt. Then, when they're old enough to decide for themselves, you will have raised the chances that they will make the right choices.

Then, there's everyone else. You may have other family, friends or roommates who share your living space. While there may be some awkward moments at first, this will be a breeze compared to the challenges you will face in the first two categories of relationships.

Certainly, you should offer to help them understand the incredible benefits of the diet you have adopted. But if they're not interested, just pretend that you are living alone as far as eating is concerned. Quietly, go about taking care of your own needs and never criticize them. If they ever want your help or advice, they will ask for it.

One final word on relationships. If you're fortunate enough to have a spouse or life partner who greatly enjoys eating the same way you do, you'll find that it can really be a lot of fun and may even be instrumental in taking your relationship to a whole new level.

27

CANCER, CLIMATE CHANGE AND WORLD HUNGER

By J. Morris Hicks

We lumped these three monster problems together because they are widely recognized as the three most serious issues facing humanity--and they all share a common cause and cure. Cancer is the most-feared of all diseases, climate change exacerbates all of the other environmental issues and world hunger is an ever worsening problem--a stark reminder of the staggering inadequacy of our global feeding model. Let's take a look at each one of these monster problems:

1. Cancer. If only our mainstream authorities would heed the game-changing scientific and clinical findings of T. Colin Campbell, PhD and John Kelly, MD in the two incredibly revealing books shown below, cancer could cease to be our most-feared disease.

Dr. Campbell provided the scientific foundation in the early nineties and presented his compelling findings in his best-selling 2005 book, *The China Study*. The most alarming information about cancer is that it was strongly associated with the consumption of animal protein. In the lab,

Campbell was able to "turn cancer on and off," simply by adjusting the level of animal protein in the diet up or down. (Protein from plants did not have this effect.)

Long before getting to know Colin Campbell, Dr. Kelly read *The China Study* and decided to test out the findings on his cancer patients in Ireland. The results were astounding. By avoiding animal-based foods, almost every patient in many dozens of cases was able to slow, arrest or reverse their disease.

In 2014, he went public with their stories in his powerful book shown here alongside his "source" book by Dr. Campbell. These two books appear on our Reading List in Chapter 33, and I encourage you (and your doctor) to read them both.

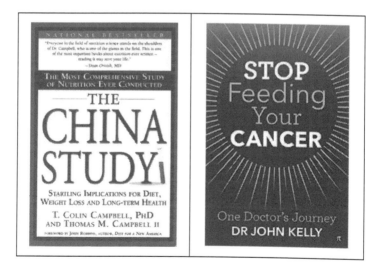

In a nutshell, Dr. Kelly has now demonstrated, with human subjects, the same remarkable facts about animal protein and cancer that Dr. Campbell observed in laboratory animals several decades ago.

Hopefully, the entire world will soon learn of the role of diet in promoting or repressing cancer. So far, the authorities in our prominent schools of medicine and nutrition have been disturbingly uninterested. From an online review of Dr. Kelly's book:

> "What Kelly has to say about the medical profession, dominated by consultants who rarely look beyond their own highly specialized areas, is telling.

> But it is his exposure of the refusal of specialists to take on board this new way of treating cancer--or even to consider it--that makes this such an important book."

This is Earth-shattering indeed—and ironic; that our *most revered* nutrient has been found found guilty of promoting our *most feared* disease.

2. Climate Change is an equally frustrating problem. A giant U.N. study, "Livestock's Long Shadow," reported in 2006 that the raising of animals for our dinner tables accounted for 18% of human-induced greenhouse gases (GHG)--more than all of the cars, trucks, buses, trains and airplanes in the world. Yet the silence has been deafening from the world's most prominent authorities.

Later, two World Bank environmental specialists, Robert Goodland and Jeff Anhang, noted that the 2006 U.N. numbers had not accounted for several significant factors. After undertaking a more unbiased and inclusive approach to the research, they reported that livestock accounted for "at least 51%" of all human-induced GHG. (For the full report, search "Goodland Anhang" on worldwatch.org.)

Of course, 51% would mean that livestock causes more global warming than all other causes combined. Yet, the frustrating silence from the authorities continues. Even the prominent environmental groups hardly even mention it, because identifying themselves as possibly being "anti-meat" would be harmful to their fundraising. Their silence on such a crucial topic is unconscionable.

3. Finally, there's world hunger. One billion people won't get enough to eat today and 20,000 children will starve to death. This is a topic that has made the headlines for almost a century. Global leaders talk about it and charitable organizations work to alleviate the suffering of the victims, but once again, no one in authority is addressing the number one cause.

Simply stated, in the developed world, we are "eating the wrong food." It all boils down to 3rd grade arithmetic. We only have enough land and water to feed the Typical Western Diet to less than half of the world's current population.

You see, on a per calorie basis, it takes over ten times as much land and water to produce animal-based foods compared to plant-based. So how have we kept up with growing demand? We've been destroying an average of thirty million acres of rainforest every year since 1970.

There are currently over two billion people whose diet consists of some form of meat, dairy, eggs and/or fish every day. And we're adding millions more each year. This is a deadly trend that must be addressed soon.

Cancer, climate change and world hunger. Amazingly, the primary cause and the best possible solution for all three is one and the same--our food choices. By simply replacing most of our animal-based foods with whole plants, we can take a giant step toward conquering all three of these monster problems in our world.

28

LOVE IS A FAR BETTER MOTIVATOR THAN FEAR

By Dr. Kerry Graff

I had the good fortune to hear Dr. Dean Ornish speak at the American College of Lifestyle Medicine conference in the fall of 2014. Impressively, he was the first physician to clinically demonstrate reversal of heart disease using lifestyle. His work is so extensive and so credible that his program was approved by Congress for Medicare reimbursement. As of this writing, it is the only such program with this distinction.

The title of Dr. Ornish's talk that day was *"The Power of Lifestyle Changes, Social Networks and Love."* He brought to my attention another great failing of my profession—the fact that physicians try to motivate patients through fear, and that fear is a poor motivator in the long run.

Sure, I've had patients quit smoking and start exercising and eating healthier right after their heart attacks, scared to death about having another. However, six months down the line, most were back to their bad habits. Although fear is an excellent motivator immediately following a life-threatening event, it is too uncomfortable for us to stay in that mindset for very long. Imagine if you motivated yourself to stick with your new healthier lifestyle only by concentrating on what horrible things might happen to you if you didn't. I'm sorry, but that doesn't sound like a life worth living.

We need to transition from thinking in terms of what bad things are going to happen if we don't change to focusing instead on what good things will happen if we do. This process is called "cognitive reframing" and it is crucial for any lasting lifestyle change. Let me take you through a personal example.

I was pre-diabetic before I adopted a whole food, plant-based diet. Initially I was motivated by fear, knowing the huge health implications of being diabetic.

> **FEAR Response**: "I don't want to become diabetic!"

> But soon after adopting a 4Leaf diet, I changed my outlook to one of love.

> **LOVE Response**: "I love the way I feel when I eat this way! I have so much more energy and enjoy life so much more than I did before. I can't wait to raft down the Grand Canyon with my kids!"

Both of these types of responses keep me motivated to stay on a healthy path, but I focus on the *Love Response* because it makes me feel happy and I don't focus on the *Fear Response* because it makes me feel scared. For my mental health, happy is much better than scared!

Please take a minute and jot down some things you would like to do in the future with your good health:

_____
_____
_____
_____

The next time a choice comes up as to what you will eat (and it will at least three times a day!), focus on making your choice from a place of love.

> For example: "I am going to eat vegetable soup rather than a hamburger for lunch because I want to: dance at my granddaughter's wedding, celebrate my 50th anniversary with a trip to Hawaii, or volunteer in El Salvador when I retire."

I don't know what it is that you love. But you do. Use it as your motivation!

Love and Fear on a Global Scale. Throughout this book, Jim and I have described social and environmental disasters that are likely to occur unless a whole lot of humans move to a plant-based diet quickly. Some might say that that qualifies as a "fear response" instead of one driven by LOVE.

If you are feeling some fear right now about the future of humanity, we have done our job to make you aware of what is truly at stake here, in addition to your personal health. Hopefully, you are now also aware that YOU CAN MAKE A DIFFERENCE with regard to really big issues like climate change and world hunger just by changing to a plant-based diet.

Instead of focusing on your fear for humanity's future, turn to what you love and what you can do to help.

29

THE "BRAIN-LOCKING" PROTEIN MYTH

By J. Morris Hicks

Exactly what is that myth? The widespread belief in the developed world that we all *need* to eat animal protein to be healthy. Nothing could be further from the truth--yet that *myth* is alive and well, and we're running out of time to dispel it. Here's the way I see it.

Because of the mistaken, yet almost ubiquitous, belief about our "most revered" nutrient, incredibly powerful solutions to our health, hunger and sustainability crises don't even make it to the table for consideration. For this reason, I consider the *protein myth* to be the most serious roadblock in the history of humankind.

For if we cannot take the "animal out of the equation" when it comes to feeding humans, we will never learn to live in harmony with nature--thereby placing the future of our civilization (and even our species) in severe jeopardy.

Urgency of Climate Change. As mentioned earlier, World Bank climate specialists reported in 2009 that the raising of livestock for human consumption is responsible for at least 51% of all human-induced greenhouse gasses. That means that our love affair with eating meat and dairy at almost every meal is by far the leading cause of climate change--indeed, it's larger than all other causes combined. And it's also the only cause that can be addressed and reduced quickly.

But sadly, the minds of our leaders are *locked* and thereby incapable of accepting, understanding and acting on this world-saving information. So, before we can enlist the support of the best and the brightest to get serious about helping us move toward that plant-based diet, we must first dispel the *protein myth* that is believed by almost everyone. And, as we do, we shall free up those brilliant minds--releasing them to address global issues by creating plant-based solutions beyond our wildest dreams.

Dispelling the *protein myth*. I feel that our best chance to change the public awareness quickly enough to make a difference is to undertake a massive, multi-faceted, privately funded, professionally managed global awareness campaign. As we begin to work on the demand side of the equation, millions of people around the world will begin choosing more plants in their diet after hearing this message enough times from reputable, highly-respected individuals and organizations. Here is the message we want the entire world to hear:

> We do not NEED to eat animal protein to be healthy. That has been proven clinically and scientifically with tons of evidence--showing that animal-based foods actually promote most chronic diseases, including cancer. On the other hand, with enough whole, plant-based foods in our diet, we can reverse or cure most of those diseases.
>
> More importantly, the widespread raising of animals for our dinner tables is grossly unsustainable, requiring over ten times as much land, water and energy as do plant-based foods. Continuing to recklessly waste those finite

> natural resources will ultimately destroy the ecosystem that sustains us. The answer is simple—all we have to do is eat a lot more plants and a lot fewer animals. Our future as a species depends on it.

As people everywhere heed that message and begin to learn the cold hard facts about their food choices, hundreds of millions will start replacing most, if not all, of their animal-based calories with healthier and "greener," plant-based alternatives. By working on the demand side of the equation, markets will quickly respond to those food choices, people will begin getting healthier, the cost of healthcare will plummet, water will become more plentiful, trees can be planted on the freed-up land and our fragile ecosystem will begin to heal.

Eventually, we must also deal with overpopulation, over-consumption and the excessive burning of fossil fuels--but those tasks will take many decades, if not centuries. Taking urgent action now with our food choices can possibly buy us the time we need to address them all.

Leadership. Like almost everything else, this process begins with leadership. Just one powerful, globally recognized leader with a reputation for integrity and care for the environment can make this happen. Once fully enlightened, he or she can quickly recruit other leaders and secure the financial resources that will be needed for swift action around the world.

You can help by adopting a plant-based diet yourself and by influencing others to do the same. As more people embrace this powerful diet-style, prominent leaders will eventually get involved and urgently take it to the next level. If you know of any powerful leaders who might be interested in saving our civilization, please refer them to me at jmh@4leafglobal.com.

30

PATIENT NOW ON PATH TO VIBRANT HEALTH

By Dr. Kerry Graff

KG: "So, it's been about a month since our last visit. How are things going?"

TM: "Great. Well, mostly. Scoring 24 (3Leaf level) pretty consistently on the 4Leaf Survey, I feel great except I get really gassy from the beans, so I have been limiting them. I'm doing yoga after work, including the relaxation part, with my wife and we both love that. I feel a lot less stressed in the evenings and even while I'm at work. I'm drinking more water, and usually keeping my wine to two a day. The after dinner TLC part was the BEST suggestion-- and I'm not talking about coffee or tea! Since I changed my diet, that is working much better. I had thought that I was just getting older."

KG: "Yes, getting the inflammation out of the arteries by cutting the oil definitely helps with blood flow and sex life! Glad all of that is going so well. As for the gassiness, over time the bacteria in your gut will shift to handle beans better, but in the short run, you can take Beano. If you are cooking your beans, adding kombu (a seaweed vegetable) while they are cooking helps to break them down so they cause less gas. Where are you losing points on the survey?"

TM: "Well, when we go over to visit friends or family, I don't feel comfortable telling them about my new way of eating so I just eat what they have. I am still drinking two glasses of wine a day so I lose a few sugar points. It isn't so much that I'm losing points, though, it's that I don't score high enough in the whole grain, bean and potato category. I eat a lot of whole grains, but they are in bread or pasta so they don't count."

KG: "I know how uncomfortable it feels to tell your hosts you are on a specific diet. I feel like I'm inconveniencing people and they won't invite me back! One of the tricks I've learned is to offer to bring something you know you can eat and, if they say don't bother, I bring it anyway! I also eat something healthy before I go, so I'm not starving. I've found it helpful to say why I'm eating this way--what my specific health issues are that prompted me to change and the success that I've had. Of course, you have to feel comfortable with your hosts to do that.

A number of people at social gatherings have changed to eating this way after I talk to them about why I did it, so you may help other people get healthier too. You can also just say that your doctor has you following this diet and blame me. I don't have to eat dinner with them! And I cut myself some slack when I'm eating at someone else's home. Food is an integral part of bonding with people and those connections are really important.

I try to eat especially healthy the rest of the day and cheat as little as I can at the meal to stay close to 4Leaf but still keep the peace. If I only eat at a 3Leaf level that day, so be it. It doesn't happen that often."

TM: "Good suggestions. I'll try those."

KG: "As for eating the processed whole grains, rather than the whole grains themselves, do you think having additional recipes might help?"

TM: "Well, two of the staple recipes we have been making are veggie pizza on whole wheat crust and veggies over whole wheat pasta. If we had some other recipes that used the whole grains rather than the processed versions, that would help."

KG: "I have a couple of whole food, plant-based cookbooks in the office you can check out. If you like one of them, you can buy it. My personal favorite is the *Oh She Glows* cookbook, but you would need to eliminate the oil, which is easy enough to do. The recipes turn out fine without it."

Another month later

TM: "I'm eating 4Leaf level just about every day! Is my bloodwork in? It's got to be good!"

KG: "Yes it is in, and yes it looks way better! Your total cholesterol is down to 220. It was 272. Your LDL is down to 128. It was 177. And your triglycerides are down to 118 from 222."

TM: "So does this mean I don't have the genetic cholesterol problem?"

KG: "Well, most people who are eating at the 4Leaf level have cholesterol levels lower than yours. So I think you do have a genetic predisposition to higher levels. But your diet had a huge impact on your numbers, and you have substantially reduced your risk with the diet changes you made. You are now hitting the guideline numbers we like to see."

TM: "Should I go on cholesterol lowering medication in addition? Would that further lower my risk?'

KG: "I would not recommend that. Medication comes with risks and side effects and I don't believe that the potential benefits of further cholesterol reduction outweigh the risks from the medication in your case since you are hitting the guideline levels."

TM: "If I go on the medication, can I go back to eating whatever I want?"

KG: "You can always do whatever you want because what you eat is your personal choice. But think back to the study by Dr. Esselstyn in *Forks Over Knives*. The folks that stuck with the diet did great. Those that didn't, and received medications and the best that modern medicine had to offer at one of the best institutions in the world, did poorly by comparison--even when their cholesterol levels looked good. Medical intervention, including cholesterol-lowering medication, is a poor substitute for an optimal diet."

TM: "Well, I feel so much better that I don't want to come off the diet anyway. I have tons of energy, my gut doesn't hurt anymore, I've lost the extra 15 pounds I was carrying, I haven't had any more kidney stones and my sex life is awesome. It does take more time and planning, but it's worth it. It's my life!"

It's my life! Does it get any better than that?

31

SUSTAINABILITY
IS PARAMOUNT

By J. Morris Hicks

In the future, things that we value most like family, health, freedom, peace, wealth, friends and happiness--will not exist without sustainability. In other words, if we don't learn how to live in harmony with nature, life will be nothing more than a hell on Earth for those few of us who manage to survive.

Many scientists now agree that Mother Nature cannot sustain the way we are living for very much longer. One of those scientists is Marcelo Gleiser, PhD, professor of natural philosophy, physics and astronomy at Dartmouth. Shortly before this book was published in the summer of 2015, his article entitled, "The High Price of What We Eat," was posted on npr.org. His conclusion:

> "Yes, meat tastes good. But we have to start asking ourselves how long we are going to ignore what is obvious--that our meat-eating culture is not environmentally sustainable. We've moved far from our Paleolithic ancestors. It's time our diet follows our cultural advances."

In addition to the way we eat, there are three other primary elements of our grossly unsustainable lifestyle. Let's recap all four:

1. Overpopulation. Having exploded from one billion to over seven billion in just 200 years, we continue to add almost a million people every four days.

2. Overconsumption. Our entire global economy is based on maximizing the consumption of "stuff" in a world of finite resources.

3. Our dependence on fossil fuels. One of the leading drivers of global warming, it is a direct result of the first two problems on this list.

4. The way we eat. Requiring over ten times as much land, water and energy (per calorie) than plant-based foods, our wildly popular Typical Western Diet is grossly unsustainable and MUST be changed.

Since it will take many decades, if not centuries, to address the first three issues, our only remaining option is to change the way we eat. Switching from the Typical Western Diet to one consisting of mostly whole, plant-based foods offers us a HUGE opportunity to begin solving our overall sustainability nightmare.

As people everywhere begin to learn the whole truth about their food choices, millions will start replacing most, if not all, of their animal-based calories with healthier and "greener," plant-based alternatives.

Some might ask, "What would happen to the billions of "food animals" alive today and would there be enough plant-based foods to go around if everyone tried to make the change too quickly?" The simple answer is that as demand drops for animal-based foods, there will be fewer animals produced each year. In the ensuing years, the entire population of "food animals" will continue to dwindle—as the era of the widespread suffering of billions of animals for our dinner plates gradually comes to an end.

What about having enough plant-based foods to go around if hundreds of millions of people tried to make the change too quickly? The short answer is that major behavior change never happens that rapidly for large populations. And, as a business man, I am totally confident that our free-market system will respond as quickly as necessary to meet the rapidly growing demand for more health promoting, world-changing, plant-based foods.

As we begin replacing most of our animal-based calories with whole, plant-based alternatives, many wonderful things will happen. As we become healthier and the cost of healthcare plummets, we'll also be taking the best possible action for our environment. Is it any surprise that Mother Nature designed it that way?

What else can YOU do?

Eat organically when you can. Currently, non-organic farming uses huge amounts of pesticides, known to be harmful to humans as well as insects and weeds. Particularly concerning are genetically modified organisms (GMOs), which are designed to either generate their own pesticides within the plant or withstand massive external application of pesticide--not healthy for us or the planet. The safety data of GMOs is extremely limited, despite being a multi-billion dollar business.

Eating organically grown food significantly reduces the amount of pesticide you ingest, although it doesn't completely eliminate exposure. Even organic foods can have some residual pesticide from contaminated water or land or from adjacent farms that do not use organic farming techniques. Do yourself and the planet a favor, buy organic when you can.

Eat locally grown produce if possible. Strawberries in January are a treat, but shipping them thousands of miles generates a lot of greenhouse gases. You will have much less environmental impact if you eat what is grown in your own backyard--literally! Growing food yourself is a wonderful way to really connect with what you eat and is a particularly effective way to get kids enthusiastic about eating vegetables.

Community Supported Agriculture (CSA) is another great way to eat locally grown food. When you join a CSA, you are buying a "share" of the farmer's crop for the season. Each week, you will get an assortment of just-picked fruits and vegetables for an affordable price. You will likely get some vegetables you have never heard of before— providing an opportunity to learn how to prepare something new.

Farmer's markets are another great option. Compared to a CSA, a farmer's market will give you more choice over what you buy and how often.

The Bottom Line. The future of our civilization and our species lies in our hands, and the positive actions of every single individual can help. Sadly, the citizens of Easter Island didn't realize that their lifestyle was unsustainable until it was too late. Hopefully, their story, covered in the next chapter, will help motivate us to take swift action to save our ecosystem NOW.

32

PROFOUND LESSONS FROM EASTER ISLAND

By J. Morris Hicks

It's extremely important that we all learn from what happened there and that we make sure that history doesn't repeat itself on the finite space where we all live today-- planet Earth. So what happened on Easter Island?

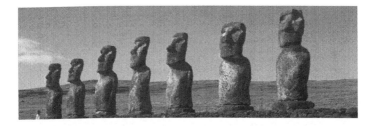

A small island (About 63 square miles) located 2300 miles off the coast of Chile in the South Pacific, the human settlers (Rapa Nui) are believed to have arrived by boat from Polynesia around 400 A.D. That's when they began to take charge of this tropical paradise that it took Mother Nature billions of years to build.

During the next one thousand years, the Rapa Nui's population exploded to around 15,000, and evidence of a fairly advanced civilization can be found there today. From the size, weight and complexity of the giant stone statues that they built and placed around the island, we know that the Rapa Nui were most certainly an intelligent and industrious group of people with a sophisticated hierarchy of leadership. (Almost 900 of those giant statues, called Moai, were found—some weighing as much as 80 tons.)

But that thriving civilization was doomed, collapsing prior to the arrival of Dutch explorers on Easter Sunday (hence, the name of the island) in 1722. That's when they found only about 2,000 remaining humans—all of them just trying to stay alive. They were the last victims of a thriving civilization that collapsed due to its inability to connect their own behavior to the demise of the ecosystem that sustained them.

Prior to the arrival of the Rapa Nui around 400 A.D., the island had been almost completely wooded with palm trees and was home to thousands of species of birds and insects. Almost all of them went extinct during the first 1,000 years of human occupation. And the humans were well on their way to becoming extinct when the Dutch arrived.

It all started with deforestation as thousands of trees were cut to make room for settlements and to provide wood for boats (needed for fishing) and shelters for the people. Without knowing the results of their folly, the Rapa Nui were depleting the island's finite resources, which led to the demise of the fragile ecosystem that sustained life there. Before they knew what was happening, it was too late.

Tragically, that's exactly what's happening today on our *Easter Island*, planet Earth. And once again, deforestation is a big part of it. Averaging thirty million acres of rainforest destroyed per year since 1970, we're destroying the "lungs of the Earth" in the process. Richard Oppenlander reported in *Comfortably Unaware* that a staggering 70% of that rainforest loss was for the raising of livestock.

When I talk about Easter Island in my presentations, I begin with two slides. The first shows a lush tropical island that it took nature billions of years to create. The second one shows how it looked after just one thousand years of human stewardship--a barren landscape. Consider this: If the four billion years of life on Earth were crammed into just one year, the human occupation of Easter Island lasted just the last ten seconds of that year--a mere blink in the eye of history.

Once again, we humans are systematically taking over a much larger amount of limited space--the entire globe. We are rapidly using up our finite resources to feed ourselves and to produce a steadily increasing amount of stuff for us to consume. And, it's not just the rainforest that's in jeopardy. It's our water supply, the biodiversity of our ecosystem, the quality of our air and more.

From a January 2015 *Washington Post* article entitled, "Human activity has pushed Earth beyond planetary boundaries."

> "At the rate things are going, the Earth in the coming decades could cease to be a "safe operating space" for human beings. That is the conclusion of a new paper published Thursday in the journal *Science* by 18 researchers trying to gauge the breaking points in the natural world."

The paper contends that we have already crossed four *planetary boundaries*: the extinction rate, deforestation, the level of carbon dioxide in the atmosphere and the flow of nitrogen and phosphorous (used on land as fertilizer) into the ocean.

As I read the article, I was reminded of a terrifying factoid mentioned in the 2009 PPR-produced documentary, HOME: "We humans have inflicted more damage on the fragile harmony of nature in just the last fifty years than all previous generations of humans combined for the 200,000 years since we emerged as a species."

To put that in perspective, fifty years would be just the last one-half second of the imaginary year (of life on Earth) mentioned earlier.

And although the depletion of our finite resources continues to worsen, none of our global leaders are talking about this terrifying "big picture," much less organizing emergency initiatives to reverse this deadly trend while we still have time. Unfortunately, our top leaders are frequently quoted as saying that life has never been better than it is now: fewer epidemics, less infant death, more wealth, better quality of life, etc.

Sadly, that's probably what the Rapa Nui were saying as they passed critical tipping points with regards to their own fragile ecosystem. But we still have hope. And we have the knowledge and the resources to turn that hope into reality.

Taking urgent action now with our food choices can buy us the time we need to address other human activities that threaten our ecosystem, our civilization and our long-term viability as a species. It is the easiest, quickest and most powerful step we can take to start restoring our ecosystem.

33

A READING LIST FOR DEEPER UNDERSTANDING

By J. Morris Hicks

Kerry and I have tried to put everything into this book that you will need to get you and our planet on the pathway to vibrant health. For the past 100 years, that pathway has been somewhat of a *road less traveled*. Hopefully that will change, but for now, you're definitely in the minority. As such, you may want to arm yourself with additional facts in order to be able to more confidently present your new knowledge in the most effective way possible.

While there is enough information in this book to get you going, there is not nearly enough for you to fully understand, believe and be able to debate some of the more controversial topics involved with a movement away from an animal-based diet for humans. By reading some or all of the following books, you'll be much better prepared.

In the list of ten recommended books below, I will save *Healthy Eating, Healthy World* for last because, to a large extent, it is a "big picture" summary of the other books. I lead off with books by the three experts who influenced

President Bill Clinton to adopt a whole food, plant-based diet to reverse his heart disease. These are followed by four more books about human health and, finally, two books about global depletion and sustainability.

1. The China Study by T. Colin Campbell, PhD, (Cornell University) and Thomas M. Campbell II, MD. Published in 2005, this book laid the scientific foundation for the global plant-based movement. In its first ten years, it sold over a million copies and has influenced countless millions of people to adopt a whole food, plant-based diet.

2. Prevent and Reverse Heart Disease, by Caldwell Esselstyn, Jr., MD, Cleveland Clinic. An incredibly powerful story about how a former surgeon halted or even reversed heart disease in 100% of the patients who followed his whole food, plant-based dietary guidelines. It also has lots of heart-healthy recipes that helped all of those patients do something that all the cardiologists in the world couldn't.

3. The Spectrum, by Dean Ornish, MD. One of the most famous advocates of plant-based eating in the world, he teaches medicine at UCSF. Notably, he was the first to prove that heart disease was reversible for almost everyone with lifestyle changes and was the first to get his program approved for Medicare. He also drew a lot of attention for his participation with Sanjay Gupta in "The Last Heart Attack" special on CNN in 2011. One of Bill Clinton's consulting physicians since 1993, Dr. Ornish is a powerful force in medicine worldwide.

4. Dr. Neal Barnard's Program for Reversing Diabetes, by Neal Barnard, MD. He graduated from the George Washington School of Medicine in Washington, DC, where he later founded the *Physicians Committee for Responsible Medicine*, which he still directs. In this great book, he helps people everywhere who no longer want to "manage" their type 2 diabetes but would rather get rid of it. And he recommends the same whole food, plant-based diet that reverses heart disease and starves cancer.

5. Stop Feeding Your Cancer, by John Kelly, MD. Working as a family physician in Ireland, he tells his amazing story in this 2014 book. In it he talks about reading *The China Study* and how he decided to test its principles particularly as it relates to preventing, slowing, stopping or reversing cancer. And, like Campbell, he found that, with only one exception (which he explains), cancer stopped growing in humans when animal protein consumption was greatly reduced or eliminated.

6. The Starch Solution, by John McDougall, MD. Like the other four pioneering medical doctors featured in *Healthy Eating, Healthy World* below, John has demonstrated to the world that we should be eating a whole food, plant-based diet. An author of many books on this topic, he has no doubt helped millions of people take charge of their health—as he promotes the critical importance of starch-based foods like grains, legumes and potatoes.

7. Whole, Rethinking the Science of Nutrition, by T. Colin Campbell, PhD. Published in 2013, this book documents all of the many reasons why the field of nutritional science has gotten it all wrong when it comes to what we should be eating.

8. TEN BILLION, by Stephen Emmott, PhD, head of Computational Science for Microsoft, based in the U.K. About a one hour read, this little book describes the grossly unsustainable pathway the human species has chosen. While he doesn't talk much about the solution, he agreed with me that we'll never get it done without radically changing what we eat. I call this a book for leaders; I only wish that all of our leaders would read it-- and begin taking urgent action.

9. Comfortably Unaware, by Richard Oppenlander. In this fairly short book, he describes the single biggest problem humankind faces--the rapid and unsustainable pace with which we are depleting our finite natural resources--with land and water topping the list. Sadly, as the title implies, the world's citizens, including most of our world leaders and environmental experts, are *comfortably unaware* of the extent of the problem. Unlike most environmental authors, Oppenlander stresses the plant-based solution as the only pragmatic way for humans to return to living in harmony with nature.

10. Healthy Eating, Healthy World, by J. Morris Hicks with J. Stanfield Hicks. Rather than tell you about this book myself, I'll let my new filmmaker friend do the honors:

> "Thank you for putting together such an amazing work. In preparation for my film, I've read over fifty books related to the subject, and your book is definitely at the very top of my favorites list. You did an amazing job of compiling the best available information out there from the best experts (Campbell, McDougall, Ornish, Fuhrman, Barnard, Robbins, and others)--and explaining it in a simple, easy-to-understand way. I am very happy to have met you and feel honored to have you participating in my film!" Michal Siewierski (FoodChoicesMovie.com)

All of these books can be purchased on Amazon from the "Store" tab at 4leafprogram.com. Another good resource, containing over 900 articles on these topics, is my own personal website at hpjmh.com.

34

PROSELYTIZING NOT RECOMMENDED

By J. Morris Hicks

While writing my first book in 2010, I was living in a quaint New England village by the sea and I knew virtually all 1200 residents by sight and about half of them by name. Just before moving there in 2003, I had become curious about the optimal diet for humans. During my extensive study, I had made startling discoveries related to saving lives and preserving life itself on planet Earth. So, what should I now be telling my new friends about those discoveries?

The short answer is nothing, unless I am asked a question. So how are we supposed to spread the word about what we consider the most important topic in the history of humanity--the staggering consequences of what we eat?

First, let's remember that eating is a very important and very personal part of everyone's life. Our entire existence is centered around eating, especially our social interactions and cultural and religious traditions. The notion that our own mothers might not have known what we should be eating or that we have been feeding food to our loved ones that contributes to their ill health is a tough pill to swallow for most people. So how do you help your friends and loved ones discover the amazing truths that you have learned about food choices?

Just live your own life and always try to do what you think is right, while remembering that it's a fine line between caring and proselytizing. When someone wants to hear your opinion about diet, they will ask you a question.

My guidelines on proselytizing are similar to my thoughts about selling. No one likes to be "sold" anything. I prefer the word "marketing," which can be a subtle process of cultivating a desire to purchase something. Here's my list of behavioral guidelines on this delicate subject:

1. Never offer unsolicited advice to anyone.
2. Don't make negative comments about an unhealthy looking meal someone else is eating.
3. Never talk about health or diet with anyone unless they ask for your opinion.
4. When people do ask for information, try to keep your initial response to a minimum. If they want to know more, they will ask.
5. Try to keep delicate discussions one-on-one. If someone asks about your eating philosophy in front of a lot of people, try to offer a concise, courteous response--then offer to continue the conversation later, perhaps over a healthy meal.

So you might be thinking, "If we can't tell people about the powerful truths that we have learned, how can we make a difference?" For starters, we can follow this simple advice from Gandhi:

Be the change you want to see in the world.

The more specific answer may be different for everyone. In my case, I decided to start a blog, write a book, get some speaking engagements, create the helpful 4Leaf concept, do some corporate consulting, become an activist and start a business aimed at helping to change the global feeding model. The more energy I put into what I do, the more doors continue to open.

To summarize, I simply don't like proselytizing and I don't think other people like being on the receiving end of it. Further, I must remember that over 90% of my friends still eat meat and dairy and that I am in the very small minority. As such, I should try to minimize uncomfortable situations for all concerned. In the long run, I sincerely believe that this approach works best. Here's an example:

Recently, a yacht club friend walked up to me at a party and told me how much he liked my book, *Healthy Eating, Healthy World*. And he did so in front of several other people. This former president of Reebok then told me that the book was "simple, not too long, easy to read and compelling--without being full of zealotry."

He then added that he would be making some changes in his own diet as a result of what he had learned from the book. I simply thanked him deeply for the feedback.

The Bottom Line. We all know that food is a very personal topic for everyone. Perhaps this chapter will help in terms of how we best share our message without causing any discomfort or resentment. People are less likely to follow your example if they resent you.

35

THE "OTHER" FIVE LEAVES OF VIBRANT HEALTH

By J. Morris Hicks

We've talked a lot about vibrant health in this book--we even mentioned it in the title. Now, we need to remind you that, while the food part is extremely important, there are a few other pieces in the *vibrant health* puzzle--at least when it comes to our own health.

In addition to diet, the American College of Lifestyle Medicine refers to five fundamental elements that make or break our health: smoking, exercise, sleep, stress and love. Those other five "leaves" are listed here, beginning with the most obvious one:

Leaf #1. Don't smoke. We don't need to waste space in this book telling you all about the health problems associated with smoking. Everyone already knows that smoking is TERRIBLE for your health, so if you really want to enjoy vibrant health, don't smoke.

Nicotine is addictive and many smokers have difficulty quitting. If you are unable to quit on your own, see your doctor who can counsel you on the options available to help you overcome this addiction.

Leaf #2. Exercise regularly. The healthiest people in the world are eating the right food AND are getting plenty of exercise. So how much exercise is enough? Many experts agree that we should try to keep our bodies in motion for at least one hour a day, just about every day of the week.

Ironically, most of the healthiest people in the world don't have gym memberships. That's because, unlike most of us in the western world, they are quite active in their daily lives. But since most of us are more sedentary, we will need to have a specific plan to get the exercise our bodies need to thrive.

Your exercise regimen should include both aerobic activity (getting and keeping your heart rate up) and strength training. These can be combined in the same activity if the aerobic activity is weight bearing (you are supporting your weight while you are doing the activity). Examples of this are running and playing tennis.

If you do non-weight bearing exercise, such as biking or swimming, for the aerobic component, you should incorporate a separate strengthening activity, like lifting small weights. Consider joining a fitness center or hiring a personal trainer if this is foreign territory for you. (See Appendix G for my own personal exercise routine.)

Leaf #3. Get adequate sleep. This is an area where people think that they can cut corners. Forget it! Getting adequate sleep is very important. The good news is that once you begin eating mostly whole, plant-based foods and exercising regularly, you will likely be sleeping much better.

How much sleep should you be getting? From the website of the National Sleep Foundation:

> "Sleep experts recommend a range of seven to nine hours of sleep for the average adult. While sleep patterns change as we age, the amount of sleep we need generally does not. Older people may wake more frequently through the night and may actually get less nighttime sleep, but their sleep need is no less than younger adults."

Sleeping more than your body needs is not good for you, either. Get to know how many hours of sleep you need to function at your best, and then make it a point to get the right amount.

Leaf #4. Manage stress well. Sure, it would be nice to have a stress-free life, but that is just not going to happen. And it would be pretty boring too. Bad things cause stress, but some of the very best things in life come with stress too--like getting married to the most wonderful partner, or having a baby or writing the book you've always dreamed of authoring.

Almost all of our stress comes from thinking about unpleasant things from the past or what unpleasant things might happen in the future. Very rarely is the stress coming from what is happening *right now*. So one of the most effective ways to manage stress is to bring your mental focus back to the current moment.

This is called Mindfulness, and there are many ways to do this: meditation, body scanning, yoga, poetry, music and many others. Find ways to cultivate Mindfulness in your daily life and you will find that you respond to life with greater ease and joy, no matter the situation.

Leaf #5. Find what you love. By that, I am talking about discovering your passion or your sense of purpose. This one definitely means different things to different people. Some people find it in their work, others find it in their church or charitable causes. It doesn't matter what it is as long as it gets you motivated and provides you with that warm, satisfying feeling of making a difference.

I recently saw this quote by a man in his eighties: "Everyone I know that is over 80 is either still working or is dead." The point is that we all seem to function better, have a more positive attitude and enjoy greater happiness if we have people to see, things to do and places to go. Life just seems to be so much more fulfilling if you've found your passion and are now on a mission.

It took me 58 years to find my passion and I plan to work on that passion diligently for the rest of my life. In my case, I simply got curious about the optimal diet for humans in November of 2002. Ten thousand hours of study and work later, I now have a new, highly-satisfying, never-ending career.

For me, it's all about doing my best to help people everywhere embrace a whole food, plant-based diet to promote health, hope and harmony on Planet Earth. I sincerely believe that there has never been anything more important in the history of humanity--and I absolutely love what I do.

36

NEW WORLD OF HARMONY

By J. Morris Hicks

Imagine for a moment that almost everyone in the world is already eating a plant-based diet. That's right--the billions of farm animals that we once raised for our dinner tables no longer exist. All the great chefs and fine restaurants of the world are focused totally on plant-based dining and are written up in the Michelin and Zagat guides everywhere.

Not only are people raving about the food, chronic disease is almost non-existent and the cost of healthcare in the USA has plummeted to record low levels--now hovering around 4% of the GDP, down sharply from the record of almost 20%.

Prominent medical schools have converted from "disease management" to health promotion and most of the medical costs now are for things like prenatal services, injury repair and cosmetic surgery. Screening tests for cancer are no longer needed since the incidence of that killer disease has shrunk to near zero.

There is enough food and fresh water for everyone on the planet and we are now only using natural resources at a responsible rate that allows Mother Nature to continuously replace them. The population has stabilized at a sustainable number and we have ended our dependence on fossil fuels.

There is widespread peace and a better quality of life throughout the world as the enormous funds that were formerly spent on healthcare, highly inefficient foods and wars--are now devoted primarily to the complete elimination of world hunger, poverty and illiteracy. The world is once again a place of near complete harmony.

And it all began with a rapid shift from animal-based foods to plant-based foods. But that transformation didn't get any real traction until enough courageous medical professionals embraced the incredible power of whole, plant-based foods to prevent and reverse disease---and then started enthusiastically promoting it to their patients.

One practitioner who has done just that is Dr. Kerry Graff, who started making big changes in her family medicine practice long before she knew how she was going to make it work from a financial standpoint. She just started helping people get healthy and the ensuing feeling of joy kept her going. While writing this chapter, I just heard from her today with this text message:

"Just saw a patient who went from a total cholesterol of 340 to 195 on 4Leaf. She feels fantastic! She looks amazing, too." ☺

So how do we get serious traction in the mainstream medical community? In the next (and final) chapter, Dr. Graff takes a powerful first step. She courageously makes a written appeal to all of her fellow physicians to join the growing global movement to replace "disease care" with true "health care."

37

CALLING ALL DOCTORS

By Dr. Kerry Graff

After first learning the powerful truths about food, many people are motivated (for a variety of reasons) to change their diets immediately--until they visit with their physician. Unfortunately, that's when they are far more likely to hear words of caution than encouragement.

That's because most physicians are still eating some version of the Typical Western Diet themselves, and thinking that pills and procedures will fix the diseases they believe are caused by genes and bad luck. After all, they are just doing what they were trained to do.

Patients asking about whole food, plant-based diets today may very well know more about health-promoting nutrition than the doctors from whom they are seeking advice. This is not acceptable, but it is our current reality. And it's not the fault of the innocent physicians.

Even if the physician is aware of the profound health benefits of a plant-based diet, it is unlikely that he or she would recommend it to patients if unwilling or unable to adopt it personally. We are considered by our patients to be the best resource for dietary advice, regardless of whether that status is deserved, and I would argue that physicians have a moral obligation to give our patients the best possible advice. And since the schools of medicine are not likely to drop the "pills and scalpel" mentality anytime soon, it's up to the doctors themselves to join forces and help each other, while trying to uphold our Hippocratic Oath to "First, do no harm."

As Susan Benigas of Plantrician.org says, "We can only make so much progress on our own. We simply must find a way to get mainstream medicine onboard when it comes to the incredible, health-promoting power of plant-based nutrition. For, until they embrace the benefits of a whole food, plant-based diet; and, in turn, promote patient adoption, this essential dietary shift on a broad scale will be elusive."

With the purpose of promoting that essential dietary shift, I have penned this letter to my fellow MDs and other medical practitioners. You might want to give a copy of it to your doctor.

Kerry Graff, MD
502 South Main Street, Canandaigua, NY, 14424

To: All Medical Providers
Subject: Prevent and reverse disease with optimal diet

Dear Fellow Medical Practitioners,

As medical professionals, we have the responsibility to provide our patients with the very best advice available when it comes to health. That includes advising them on what they should be eating. In fact, I would argue that dispensing sound, health-promoting dietary advice is our single most important responsibility. Why is that? Because what a patient eats matters more to their health than any pill we can prescribe or procedure we can do.

Although not yet being taught in medical schools, there now exists a mountain of evidence supporting the fact that a whole food, plant-based diet can prevent, reverse or even cure most of the chronic diseases experienced in western society. It is now crystal clear that humans should be eating far more whole plants and far less meat, dairy, eggs, fish and highly-processed foods. With that *mountain of evidence*, it is now morally imperative that we educate ourselves and our patients about these powerful nutritional truths and their monumental impact on human health.

What can this powerful diet-style can do for our patients? For starters, studies have shown that more than 95% of heart patients adopting this diet will NEVER HAVE ANOTHER CARDIAC EVENT. Type 2 diabetes can be reversed in almost all cases and cured in many. And most cancers can be prevented or halted if they have already started. The health benefits are extraordinary.

From a personal perspective, I have had the privilege of watching many of my chronically ill patients get profoundly better when they adopted this diet-style after hearing my enthusiastic recommendation. Patients are overjoyed to be regaining their health and getting off their medicines. And, after years of feeling like I was just "sticking my finger in the dike" as I prescribed pills to treat chronic diseases, I have rediscovered the joy of practicing medicine.

But what if you consider a whole food, plant-based diet to be a little…extreme? Some doctors do feel that way and, as such, may be uncomfortable recommending a diet-style to their patients that they may not be willing to adopt themselves. To me, that is a big problem.

Consider the millions of patients out there who would think that open heart surgery, colostomy or early death is much more *extreme* than eating broccoli, beans and apples. How would those patients feel if they found out that we knew about the power of diet to prevent, reverse and even cure disease, but chose not to tell them because of our own personal bias? Why should the innocent public NOT be told about this lifesaving information simply because their physician feels that it might be too extreme for him or herself personally?

As patients learn about the tremendous impact of a whole food, plant-based diet on health, some of them will enthusiastically embrace it. Others won't. But I passionately believe that it should be their choice, and that every patient should be educated so that they're equipped to make an informed decision--and offered high quality resources and support should they choose to try it. Isn't presenting it as an option when discussing prevention and treatment of disease essential for informed consent?

Imagine if we had a medication available that could prevent, reverse or cure the vast majority of chronic diseases and we didn't bother to even discuss it with our patients. Just imagine the outcry! Obviously, we would tell all of them about that new wonder drug because not doing so would be unconscionable. Dispensing sound, dietary advice for preventing and reversing disease is no different. Ultimately, the primary access vehicle for hearing the truth about the profound effect of diet on health should be the physician--whether or not that physician is willing to adopt a superior diet-style him or herself.

I believe that prescribing a whole food, plant-based diet should and will soon become the standard of care for all healthcare practitioners, regardless of specialty. In addition, while smoking status is routinely assessed at every patient visit, evaluation of dietary health is neglected. This is despite the fact that the CDC estimates that poor diet is as harmful to health as is smoking.

One of the reasons we fail to assess diet quality is because we lacked a quick tool to do so...until now. The 4Leaf Survey, composed of 12 multiple choice questions about dietary habits that can be completed by patients in under 3 minutes, is that tool. The 4Leaf score generated from the survey serves as a dietary "vital sign," indicating the healthfulness of that patient's diet. For more information on the 4Leaf Survey and other tools to improve diet, please visit 4Leafprogram.com or read the *4Leaf Guide to Vibrant Health*, which I co-authored with J. Morris Hicks.

It is time for health care providers to truly promote in our daily work these words by the founder of modern medicine, Hippocrates:

Let food be thy medicine and medicine be thy food.

Without a doubt, the process of enlightening our patients about the well-established, health-promoting and disease reversing power of plant-based nutrition is long overdue. We must urgently promote it in the medical community now, knowing that its adoption by the public will have limited success without the enthusiastic endorsement from the people patients trust most--us.

Please educate yourself on this critical topic by visiting nutritionstudies.org, plantrician.org, nutritionfacts.org or reading a few books on the topic. For abundant scientific and clinical evidence supporting the "mostly whole plant" diet style, I recommend reading *The China Study* by T. Colin Campbell, PhD and Tom Campbell, MD.

Please feel free to contact me if you would like more information or would like to discuss this further.

Sincerely, Kerry Graff, MD

P.S. In addition to being of profound importance to a person's personal health, I have come to believe that "what humans eat" is the most important topic in the history of humanity. The economic and environmental benefits of a plant-based diet are enormous.

Our highly inefficient, harmful and grossly unsustainable western diet is the primary driver of up to 80% of our cost of healthcare and practically ALL of our most serious environmental problems, including climate change. Indeed, the future of our civilization and our species is being put at risk by what we are putting on our forks and into our mouths. Luckily, the solution to all of these problems is one and the same—eating mostly whole plants. But then, it really isn't just luck, is it? For when we take care of Mother Nature, she, in turn, takes care of her own.

A Few Closing Words

Throughout this book, Jim and I have encouraged you to visit 4leafprogram.com for all the latest on the survey, the other tools, recipes, etc. That's also where you can find a printer friendly, pdf copy of the above letter--so that you can print it off and hand it to your doctor on your next visit. If you are not going to be there for awhile, you might want to send it via snail-mail.

One more thing, while reading this book, you may have found yourself wondering how we got into such a mess in the first place and why you've never heard any of this information before. Well, Jim Hicks tells the entire story in his own words in the Epilog that follows.

EPILOG

How Did All of This Happen?

By J. Morris Hicks

It is crucially important that many more people learn the very important truths about the way we eat and how it affects our health and longevity, our environment and the future of life on planet Earth. This final piece may help you understand how we got into this mess in the first place and what we must do to get back to living in harmony with nature.

In 2007, after studying the global human feeding model for five years, I suddenly realized that the rare "big picture" knowledge that I had acquired on this most crucial of topics, must be documented. At that moment, I became concerned that I might die without sharing all of these truths with my loved ones, so I immediately got busy writing.

As I pounded the keyboard of my laptop on a Delta flight from Boston to Atlanta, I was thinking to myself, "This is what I would want to tell all of my closest family and friends if I knew that I had just *Thirty Minutes to Live*," my original title for this piece. I later changed it to the less morbid, *Give Me Thirty Minutes and I'll Give You Thirty Years*. That letter to my loved ones begins here.

Dear Ones,

You may have trouble understanding and/or believing some of my message; but for now, just listen. Later, if you are interested, I urge you to do your own homework, read, study and discover for yourself the simple truth about the way all of the pieces fit together. Here's how I see it:

1. Let's begin with nature. All species were created to work together in sustainable harmony, and things worked pretty well for millions of years until just a few hundred years ago. That's when human beings started doing things that were not in harmony with nature. They began eating an unnatural diet for their species, one thing led to another and gradually things got out of control. In just the past 200 years, the human population of the world has grown from one billion to the seven billion-plus that we have today. During that period (a mere blink of history), as humans became what Mark Twain called "the infestation of planet Earth," mankind drifted far away from nature's course and created an unsustainable lifestyle that has resulted in a sad combination of global sickness, widespread starvation and a host of environmental problems throughout the world.

2. The good news is that it's not too late to repair the damage. I believe that the best place to start trying to fix this mess is by doing something about the healthcare crisis that is rapidly spreading throughout the world. Fortunately, the solution is refreshingly simple, although the process of making the change is extremely complex and difficult. A little background--we are not winning the war on cancer and heart disease is still the number one killer, while both obesity and type 2 diabetes have been on a meteoric rise for the past thirty years. What's going on here? We have gradually shifted to a diet that does not provide our body with the nutrients it needs to take care of itself; concurrently, that diet has also caused a tremendous amount of environmental damage. So, if we can just teach people how to promote their own health, a by-product of that improved lifestyle will work wonders for the environment as well.

3. Did you know that, for the most part, you can choose the level of health that you desire? Our bodies have the power to heal themselves of, or prevent, most of the disease we experience in the western world. We simply must provide them with the nutrients, the exercise, the rest and the desire in order for this miracle to happen. By choosing health, you will be able to enrich your life for as long as you may live. Our bodies were designed to function with vibrant health for our entire lives, but they must be given the right fuel for starters. Most of us put much more thought into the type of fuel that we put in our cars than we do the food we put into our bodies.

4. Your food will be your medicine. Hippocrates, known as the Father of Medicine, said thousands of years ago "First, do no harm--your food will be your medicine and your medicine will be your food." He was referring to the human body's ability to promote health provided that we feed it the right stuff. Although our doctors still take the Hippocratic Oath upon graduation from med school, today's methods of treatment bear no resemblance to the wisdom expressed by Hippocrates. What happened?

5. Today's doctors do not promote health; they treat symptoms. Unfortunately, modern medicine took the wrong road many years ago, moving away from promoting health and toward treating all diseases with drugs, surgery, radiation, chemotherapy, etc. Sadly, our medical schools do not teach future doctors how to promote health; they only teach them how to diagnose problems, and then how to prescribe treatment, which often does more harm than good. Rather than addressing the underlying cause of the problem, doctors typically prescribe drugs which are often toxic. Why don't the doctors learn to promote health? Well, you see, there is no money to be made in the medical industry by teaching millions of people how to take charge of their own health and get healthy for good.

6. Most disease results from nutritional folly. My friend, Dr. Joel Fuhrman, estimates that if everyone ate an optimal diet, we would need 90% fewer doctors. As he says, "We live in an era where the majority of Americans think that diseases strike us because of misfortune, genetics, or unknown factors beyond our control. When serious disease strikes, we run to doctors and expect them to fix us with a pill. Most people have no idea that most diseases--including cancers, heart disease, strokes and diabetes--are the result of nutritional folly and are avoidable."

7. What does he mean by nutritional folly? Most Americans eat what has become known as the Standard American Diet and it features animal products and processed foods three meals a day, 365 days a year. While humans have always craved calorie-dense foods like meat, oil and cheese, it was simply not available or affordable in great quantities until about 60 or 70 years ago. That is when a bunch of clever business people began to mass-produce and distribute those types of foods efficiently. As the average person became able to afford those foods at almost every meal, the trouble really got started. Whole populations began to experience the diseases that had previously been somewhat exclusive to the affluent class.

8. Diseases of Affluence. In the olden days, only royalty and the very rich could afford these "rich" foods and guess what? The upper class began to suffer from obesity, heart disease, type 2 diabetes, cancer, osteoporosis and other diseases that came to be known as the *diseases of affluence.*

Conversely, in populations where most people primarily ate whole, plant-based foods, those diseases have been almost non-existent--until now. With the exportation of our Standard American Diet (SAD) to Japan, China, India and other countries, those people are now experiencing surges in the diseases that are rampant in the good old USA.

9. How healthy is SAD? We have been eating this way for so long now that most people think that SAD is a pretty healthy diet and that it can be a superior diet if they simply "watch what they eat," whatever that means. The truth of the matter is that SAD contains very little nutrition and is primarily responsible for the obesity epidemic as well as the prevalence of cancers, heart disease, diabetes and stroke, just to name a few.

10. How did all of this happen and why haven't you heard of this before? Well, not knowing that these foods were unhealthy, humans started eating them because they tasted good. Over the years, food manufacturers got better at producing these foods cheaply, doctors got better at treating the diseases caused by these foods, pharmaceutical companies got better at developing drugs that relieve symptoms caused by these foods, the media has been smart enough to not say bad things about the products of its sponsors, advertisers gradually convinced the public that the unhealthy products are actually good for them and the government just tries to keep the economy going so that the politicians can get re-elected.

All of the above has worked together to create one of the sickest nations on Earth, despite the fact that our healthcare (disease care) costs are by far the highest in the world. It's really no one's fault. Most people who work in the "system" actually believe they are doing good things; they are just doing what they have been taught and are all simply trying to make a living.

11. What is the answer to solving this dilemma? The answer lies in learning the truth about nutrition. Most nutritionists, dietitians, doctors and nurses only know what they have been taught and, unfortunately, they haven't been taught the simple truth about how we can promote health with food. Luckily, the information is out there for those who take it upon themselves to learn it. You see, the healing powers of nutritional excellence have been known for a long time but they simply haven't been embraced for the many reasons listed in Point #10 above.

If you really want to learn the truth, you should start with the written works of Colin Campbell, Caldwell Esselstyn, John McDougall, Dean Ornish, Neal Barnard and Joel Fuhrman. And don't stop there, keep reading and studying until your knowledge of nutrition is solidly embedded in your life permanently. The following paragraphs cover some of the many things that you will learn about food.

12. The optimal diet for humans. Human beings are herbivores; our hands, our teeth, our intestines, indeed our entire bodies are designed to eat plants. Sure, our forefathers probably ate almost anything they could get their hands on, but that doesn't mean it was good for them. Other herbivores include animals like gorillas, elephants, horses and giraffes; all of which manage to become big and strong without the "animal protein" that most Americans truly believe they must have in order to be healthy.

In addition to the essential vitamins, minerals and phytochemicals; this natural diet provides us with the fiber that we need. It is recommended that we get at least 25 grams per day but the average American gets less than 10 grams. An optimal diet will ensure that you average between 50 and 80 grams per day--and when you do, you won't need reading material in your bathroom anymore.

13. As herbivores, the natural food for our species is whole plants. We know from a vast amount of research that the healthiest plant foods for us are those still in nature's package--whole and unrefined fruits, vegetables, grains, legumes, nuts and seeds. The gorilla in the wild eats almost nothing but raw plants. We Americans, on the other hand, get a paltry 7% of our calories from whole, plant-based foods; with the remaining 93% of our calories coming from meat, cheese, chips, sweets, sodas, fries, oils and other highly refined products with very low amounts of nutrients per calorie. Most Americans are over-fed and under-nourished; as SAD is woefully short on fiber, vitamins, minerals and phytonutrients.

14. Why traditional weight-loss diets don't work. Studies show that most diets have a 97% failure rate; only 3% of the people manage to lose weight and keep it off. So, what's the problem? Weight-loss diets are unsustainable because they lack critical nutrients and leave you continually craving more food. The answer to achieving one's ideal weight and optimal health is the adoption of a permanent diet-style based on nutritional excellence. Once you learn how to select, prepare and eat the right kinds of foods, your body will take care of the rest--without calorie counting, portion control or deprivation. How considerate of Mother Nature to make things so convenient for us.

15. What portion of our diet should be whole, plant-based foods? In nature, the ideal would be 100%; however, that is probably not practical in today's world. Experts, like Dr. Fuhrman, define the optimal diet as one where at least 80% of the calories are derived from whole, unrefined, plant-based foods. While moving from 7% to

40% of calories from these highly nutritious foods would definitely be a good move, the experts agree that in order to have the maximum protection against disease and to enjoy vibrant health your entire life, you really need to shoot for 80% or better. That will also ensure that you greatly exceed the minimum target of 25 grams per day for fiber. That alone will make a huge difference in the way your body functions.

16. Why should I shift to this plant-based diet? For me, the most important reason was health. This diet-style will protect you from diseases of affluence, provide you with vibrant health for your entire life and will very likely keep you out of the nursing home in your final years. Along the way, you will get sick less frequently, maintain a trim body without "dieting," feel more energy, have a better complexion, sleep better, enjoy better sex, have less body odor, save money on food, think more clearly, reduce your chances of developing dementia, eliminate constipation forever, minimize menstrual cramps, improve eyesight, lower blood pressure, reduce or eliminate asthma, allergies and bad breath, lower bad cholesterol, eliminate most (if not all) prescription drugs and on and on and on. And that's just a few of the *health* benefits. There are many other reasons for eating this way; read on.

17. Almost everyone claims to be an environmentalist. It's hard to find anyone these days who doesn't think that doing "green" things for the environment is a good thing. Unfortunately, just like with the nutrition issue, we haven't been told the complete truth about what causes the most environmental damage. Take global warming for example; if we took a poll regarding that issue, I would bet you that that the average American would list the gas guzzling cars and trucks as the single biggest villain because that's what was conveyed in Al Gore's 2006 movie *An Inconvenient Truth.*

Would it surprise you to know that the raising of livestock for our dinner tables causes at least 30% more global warming than ALL of transportation in the entire world combined? That data was reported by the United Nations in November of 2006, but for some strange reason, the media has never seen fit to share that little tidbit with the general public. Why not? Refer to Point #10. And the great news here is that, unlike global transportation, which would be almost impossible to reduce very much if at all (considering population growth), with the raising of livestock, it would be relatively simple to eliminate the entire industry--just by shifting to a plant-based diet. This obvious solution is never mentioned in the media because very few environmentalists understand that eliminating meat from our diets would be a good idea from a nutritional standpoint.

18. Global warming isn't the only environmental problem. There are many more--and they've gotten our attention. Everyone seems to be buying hybrid cars and recyclable bags, restricting their use of water and trying to use less electricity--but darn few are even thinking about reducing their consumption of animal foods. Maybe if they learned about the other environmental problems caused by the animal foods industry--things like water pollution, topsoil erosion, depletion of our water supply, unprecedented species extinction, destruction of the rain forests and land degradation--things would be different. The key to all of this is education--everyone must learn what is really happening or there won't be much of a planet left for the future generations that follow us.

19. World Hunger. Are you worried about how we will manage to continue feeding the planet's booming population? A little background--it took the world's human population 99,900 years to grow from about 10,000 people to two billion. Then, in just the last 100 years

(1/10,000 of the time), we added another five billion people, bringing us up to the SEVEN BILLION+ that we have today. So what kind of a job are we doing in feeding all those people? Not very well actually, considering that more than a billion people go to bed hungry every night.

Contributing to that sad state of affairs are the shortcomings of our extremely inefficient method of feeding ourselves. I am referring to the Typical Western Diet or SAD that we are now exporting throughout the world. Did you know that it takes about two football fields worth of land to feed one person SAD? Any idea how many plant-eaters you could feed on that same amount of land? Would you believe fourteen? Not only would everyone be a lot healthier, but we could feed well over ten times as many people, while doing some wonderful things for our fragile environment.

20. Pretty compelling stuff, huh? Let me get this straight; by just eating a nutritious plant-based diet, we can prevent or cure heart disease, cancer and type 2 diabetes, we can greatly improve the vibrancy of our lifelong health, we can save the environment and we can solve the age-old problem of world hunger. Why then, for God's sake, are there so few people eating this way? Does it taste bad? Is it expensive? Is it too much work?

21. The Majority Rules. Most people must think that the Typical Western Diet is a smart way to eat since over 90% of the people in the developed world are eating some version of it today. If you have heard what I have said so far, you should know by now that the TWD is a very unhealthy, inefficient, destructive and unsustainable diet. Even so, its popularity continues to grow, while only about one percent of us are eating the optimal diet, getting at least 80% of our calories from whole, unrefined plant-based foods. Why? Refer back to Point #10.

There are many barriers out there that only a solid education can tear down. Right now, most of us get all of our nutrition information from television, magazines, newspapers, the internet, our doctors, friends and relatives. The net effect of all of the above is that people who eat the optimal diet are in a very small minority and are often thought to be a little weird. Many people think that we have lost our minds and that we will soon be very ill or die due to a lack of animal protein in our diets.

22. Vegetarians get a bad rap. Be honest, what comes to mind when you think of a vegetarian? You probably don't think of gold medal winners like Carl Lewis, Edwin Moses or Dave Scott; all of whom are vegetarians. For the record, I do not refer to myself as a vegetarian. The problem with "labels" like *vegetarian* or *vegan* is that they only give people some clues about what you don't eat; they don't describe what you DO eat, and that is what's most important.

While the vast majority of my calories come from whole plant foods, on occasion I will have a bite of fish, cheese or eggs while visiting in someone's home; therefore I am not a vegetarian. So, what am I? I am simply one person who has learned the truth about nutrition and has made the decision to give my body the best possible foods that I can find. And since I ate SAD for almost sixty years, I don't want to waste too many of my calories on foods that afford me no protection but rather might damage my body. I have to think about the damage I may have done during those first 58 years.

23. When does heart disease start? Heart disease and other common western diseases start developing the day we start eating a diet that is heavy in animal-based foods and light in fresh fruits and vegetables. We have been led to believe that these diseases are a natural part of the aging process. That is simply not true. These diseases are the natural result of eating a harmful diet like the TWD. Autopsies of U.S. soldiers killed in Korea showed that almost 80% of these young men in their twenties had significant coronary artery disease--it just hadn't been diagnosed yet. The age to start eating a healthy diet is as young as you possibly can. Studies show that our diet as children is one of the best predictors of the kinds of diseases we will suffer as older adults. We also know from numerous recent studies that heart disease is reversible with a superior diet.

24. Can't imagine life without cheeseburgers? I mentioned the many barriers that prevent people from embracing the healthy diet that I have described. One of those barriers is that people simply can't imagine life without some of their favorite foods. Some say that they would rather die young than give up their bacon and eggs, burgers, steaks, lobsters, cheese, pizza, etc. People actually feel addicted to these foods and think that they cannot live without them. But, in my opinion, those addictions can be broken much easier than addictions to cocaine, nicotine, and caffeine. To be sure, they are bad habits—but habits can be broken and can be replaced with healthier ones.

25. The Joy of Eating. Let's face it; food is a very big part of everyone's life. Almost everything we do centers around some form of feeding ourselves. We eat at church socials, wine and cheese receptions, parties, business lunches, when we drink, when we smoke, when we watch TV, at sporting events, graduations, weddings, in the movies, as a bedtime snack and on and on. And we like it. We have also become accustomed to eating the same kinds of unhealthy foods for most of our lives. So how do we change?

We must become educated to the extent that we can make a real commitment to a healthier diet-style. And then, when you do that, guess what happens? You will find, as have thousands before you, that you will truly find more joy in eating than ever before. Your taste buds will change, you will savor natural flavors and it will feel good to know that your meal did not damage the environment. Further, you will never have to worry about eating too much or being overweight again--just eat all you want. Finally, not a single animal will have suffered or died so that you could have their dead flesh on your dinner plate.

26. So what about the animals? As a young boy, I worked in my dad's dairy, hog and chicken operations and found myself feeling a closeness to some of those farm animals. I also saw a few slaughterhouses and can remember them vividly to this day. I sincerely believe that if all of us were forced to spend one day a year working in a slaughterhouse, that the consumption of animal foods would take a very sharp decline. Paul McCartney says, and I agree, "If slaughterhouses had glass walls, we would all be vegetarians." Almost everyone claims to love animals, yet we casually eat animal flesh from billions of animals without any thought about the barbaric treatment and disgusting torture these animals must endure for their entire lives. We buy our nicely-packaged meats with names like sirloin steak, pork sausage, veal cutlet and we feed our children *Happy Meals*. I wonder how many children would become vegetarians at the age of six if part of the first grade included a mandatory trip to a slaughterhouse.

27. It's not going to be easy, but it's worth it. Nobody in the very small minority has ever had it easy while bucking something as wildly popular as SAD. But, that doesn't mean that we should stop trying. Once you are educated, and know for sure that you are right, you must never stop trying to promote a healthier diet for all--for your health, for the starving children, for the environment, for the critters and for your future great-grandchildren who will follow us on planet Earth.

28. If you give it four months, it's really not that hard to change. When you have become educated to the extent that you have a conviction to shift to this wonderful diet-style, I recommend that you take the *4Leaf, 4-Month Challenge.* Clean out your cupboards of the unhealthy items and remove all meat and dairy from your diet. Start putting the high-powered, nutrient-dense plant-foods in your body and see how you're feeling at the end of four months.

You may suffer a few unpleasant effects of detoxification during part of your journey, but this will pass. Just stay with it and the chances are very good that you will never want to go back to your old way of eating. Why four months? To be sure, you'll notice many benefits within weeks, but the longer you stick with it, the greater the odds that this healthy change in your diet will be permanent.

29. Give Me 30 Minutes and I'll Give You Thirty Years. You see, the average period of good health ends for most people by the time they are in their fifties or sixties. With proper nutrition, exercise and motivation, there is no reason you shouldn't enjoy vibrant health for your entire life--well into your eighties and beyond--maybe even to 105 or older.

30. Who would want to live to be 105 anyway? My answer to that question is simply this, "How about a vibrantly healthy 104 year-old who had great sex last night?" Acknowledging at my ripe old age that I still have a sense of humor.

And so, "Dear Ones,"

I pray that you will learn from this message, enjoy your life and do all that you can to leave our planet in better shape than you found it.

Once you understand how all of the pieces are connected, you will know what actions to take for your own health and for the health of the planet that supports us all.

Sincerely, Jim

> J. Morris Hicks, CEO, 4Leaf Global, LLC
> Writer. Speaker. Activist.

APPENDIX A – THE 4LEAF SURVEY
(Standard form. Enter your responses on the next page.)

1. Fresh fruit. On average, how many **daily servings** of whole, fresh fruit do you eat? (Fruit juice doesn't count; not a whole plant.)

2. Whole vegetables. On average, how many **daily servings** of whole vegetables do you eat?

3. Whole grains, legumes, potatoes. On average, how many **daily servings** of these do you eat?

4. Omega-3s. Are you getting all you need from whole, plant-based sources like flaxseeds, walnuts, and chia seeds?

5. Dairy foods. How many **days per week** do you <u>eat</u> dairy foods like cheese, yogurt, and ice cream?

6. Eggs. How many **days per week** do you either eat eggs or add them as an ingredient when cooking?

7. Cow's milk or cream. How many **days per week** do you <u>drink</u> or add to your food, like cereal, coffee, etc.?

8. Added Sugar. Are you really serious about eliminating added sugar at home and in food products that you buy?

9. White flour. Bread, pasta, cakes, cookies. How would you describe your consumption level of these foods?

10. Sweets and Salty Snacks. How would you best describe your consumption level of these foods?

11. Meat, poultry and fish. How many of your **meals per week** include any animal flesh? (beef, pork, lamb, chicken, turkey or fish)

12. Vegetable Oil. How many of your **meals per week** include any oil, like olive, canola or coconut? (All oil is 100% fat, not a whole plant.)

STANDARD SURVEY INSTRUCTIONS

Just be honest and select the "points" for the response that best describes your eating habits for each question. Then, add up your plus and minus points and calculate your score on the next page.

(Our definition of a serving = about ¼ of a plate.)

Survey Questions (Answer on top, points beneath)

	Positive Points	**From**	**#1**	**To**	**#4**
1	**Fresh Fruit**	None	1-2	3-5	6+
	Avg. servings/day	0	+6	+12	+14
2	**Whole Veggies**	None	1-2	3-5	6+
	Avg. servings/day	0	+6	+12	+14
3	**Grains/Beans**	None	1-2	3-5	6+
	Avg. servings/day	0	+6	+12	+14
4	**Omega-3s**	No	Maybe	Unsure	YES
	Getting enough?	0	0	0	+2
	Negative Points	**From**	**#5**	**To**	**#12**
5	**Dairy Foods**	Never	1-2	3-5	6-7
	Days/week eaten	0	-3	-5	-7
6	**Eggs**	Zero	1-2	3-5	6-7
	Days/week eaten	0	-2	-4	-6
7	**Milk/Cream**	None	1-2	3-5	6-7
	Days/week used	0	-1	-3	-5
8	**Added Sugar**	You bet	Fairly	Not very	No
	Seriously limiting?	0	-1	-2	-3
9	**White Flour**	Zero	Light	Med.	Heavy
	Consumption level	0	-1	-3	-5
10	**Snacks**	Minimal	Light	Med.	Heavy
	Consumption level	0	-1	-3	-5
11	**Meat/Poultry/**	0-1	2-5	6-11	12+
	Fish. Meals/week	0	-3	-6	-10
12	**Vegetable Oil**	0-1	2-5	6-11	12+
	Meals/week	0	-1	-2	-3

See complete questions on previous page.

SURVEY SCORING PROCEDURE

To calculate your 4Leaf Score, subtract your total negative points from your total positive points. That will yield your net numerical score which is converted to your "4Leaf" score using the table below.

Six Levels	Range	of	Points
4Leaf	+30	to	+44
3Leaf	+20	to	+29
2Leaf	+10	to	+19
1Leaf	0	to	+9
Better than Most	-1	to	-20
Unhealthful Diet	-21	to	-44

Confused? Take a look at this example:

    12   **Positive points**

   - 27   **Negative points**

=   **-15**   **Net points**

After subtracting your negative points from your positive points, you have a net numerical score of -15, which converts to a 4Leaf score of "Better than Most."

Compute your score now:

_____   **Positive points**

_____   **Subtract negative points**

= _____   **Net points**

My Baseline 4Leaf Score = _____

Find survey forms under "Tool Kit" at 4leafprogram.com

APPENDIX B – THE 4LEAF SURVEY DAILY REPORTING VERSION

1. Fresh fruit. How many **servings** of whole, fresh fruit did you eat today? (Do not count fruit juice; not whole plant.)

2. Whole vegetables. How many **servings** of whole vegetables did you eat today? (Do not count vegetable juice.)

3. Whole grains, legumes, and potatoes. How many **servings** of these did you eat today?

4. Omega-3s. Are you getting all you need from whole, plant-based sources like flaxseeds, walnuts, and chia seeds?

5. Dairy foods. How many of your **meals** today included dairy foods (not drinks) like cheese, yogurt, and ice cream?

6. Eggs. How many **meals** today included eggs?

7. Cow's milk or cream. How many **times** today did you <u>drink</u> these or add them to your food, cereal, coffee?

8. Added Sugar. Are you really serious about eliminating added sugar at home and in food products that you buy?

9. White Flour. Bread, pasta, cakes, cookies, etc. How would you describe your consumption level of these foods?

10. Sweets & Salty Snacks. How would you best describe your consumption level of these unhealthy foods?

11. Meat, poultry and fish. How many of your **meals** today included any animal flesh? (including fish)

12. Vegetable Oil. How many of your **meals** today included any type of oil? (Don't forget salad dressing.)

Instructions: Just be honest and select your points for each of the 12 questions. Then add up your plus and minus points. (Our definition of a serving = about ¼ of a plate)

12 Survey Questions (**Answer on top, points beneath**)

	Positive Points	**From**	**#1**	**To**	**#4**
1	**Fresh Fruit** # servings today	None 0	1-2 +6	3-5 +12	6+ +14
2	**Whole Veggies** # servings today	None 0	1-2 +6	3-5 +12	6+ +14
3	**Grains/Beans** # servings today	None 0	1-2 +6	3-5 +12	6+ +14
4	**Omega-3s.** Getting enough?	No 0	Maybe 0	Not sure 0	YES +2
	Negative Points	**From**	**#5**	**To**	**#12**
5	**Dairy Foods** In # meals today	Never 0	1 -3	2 -5	3 -7
6	**Eggs** In # meals today	Zero 0	1 -2	2 -4	3 -6
7	**Milk/Cream** # times today	None 0	1 -1	2 -3	3+ -5
8	**Added Sugar** Seriously limiting?	You bet 0	Fairly -1	Not very -2	No -3
9	**White Flour** Consumption level	Zero 0	Light -1	Med. -3	Heavy -5
10	**Snacks** Consumption level	Minimal 0	Light -1	Med. -3	Heavy -5
11	**Meat/Poultry/ Fish.** Meals today	0-1 0	1 -3	2 -6	3 -10
12	**Vegetable Oil** Meals today	0-1 0	1 -1	2 -2	3 -3

See previous appendix for scoring procedures.
Find survey forms at "Tool Kit" at 4leafprogram.com.

APPENDIX C -- GOING 4LEAF SERIES
WEEK 1: PLANNING
By Dr. Kerry Graff

Week 1- Game Plan. This week you are going to:

1. Figure out what your weekly plan will be for meal planning, food shopping and batch cooking.
2. Decide what you want to eat for your routine breakfast.
3. Decide what 4Leaf snacks you would like to have on hand at all times.
4. Toss or give away (family, friends, local food bank or shelter) all of your unhealthy breakfast foods and snacks.

Eating 4Leaf has tremendous benefits, but it does require some advance planning for what you ARE going to be eating. Because it's a lot easier to eat 4Leaf when you are preparing your own food, we're going to concentrate on the meals you prepare yourself. For how to handle eating at social gatherings and while traveling, see Chapter 15 on Eating Outside the Home.

Making your plan. You will need to figure out when in your weekly schedule you are going to create a meal plan and shopping list, when you are going to shop and when you are going to do your batch cooking. For example, I have more time during the weekend than during the week, so I usually do my meal planning and shopping on Saturday and do some batch cooking on Sunday.

Many people have schedules like mine and this will work well for them. If you have a different schedule or are away a lot on the weekends, you will need to figure out the best way to incorporate these tasks into your week. THIS IS

INCREDIBLY IMPORTANT! If you don't have a workable plan for picking out what you are going to be eating as well as when you will buy and cook your food, it is highly unlikely you that will be successful in reaching the 4Leaf level of eating.

Give this some serious thought and map out a plan, knowing that it is not set in stone. You can always try a different plan if the one you start out with is unworkable, or you can tweak it if your schedule is going to be different for a particular week.

Decide when each week you will:

- Create a meal plan and shopping list
- Grocery shop
- Cook

One of the things I hear frequently from patients is "I'm too busy to meal plan and cook!" I don't buy it.

Seriously, there is nothing more important in life than your health. And there is nothing more important to the health of you and your family than what all of you eat. So you need to move planning and preparing healthy meals near the top of your "to do" list, right after breathing.

I work full time, have my kids half-time, am president of my church board, am writing this book and I still make time to meal plan, shop and cook 4Leaf (and even sleep 8 hours a night and get some exercise in too!). Granted, my life is full to the gills, but I do it. You can too.

My guess is you won't have to quit your job or have to tell your son that he can't play hockey to make 4Leaf meals happen at your house. How much time do you spend watching TV or surfing the net? If there really is no option but to choose between healthy food for your family or your son playing hockey, then hockey, not healthy eating, should be the thing to go.

And once you start eating 4Leaf, your energy level will go up significantly. You can channel some of that energy back into your new 4Leaf lifestyle.

IMPORTANT. Before you start Week 2, get rid of ALL the junk you used to eat for breakfast and ALL of your unhealthy snacks like chips, candy and ice cream. I am really serious about this! (See Chapter 14 on Contraband, beginning on page 48.)

One more tip during your planning stage: Take "before" pictures, weigh yourself and set aside a little money for some new clothes. After a few weeks on your new 4Leaf regime, you are going to like how your body looks and feels.

APPENDIX D -- GOING 4LEAF SERIES
WEEK 2: BREAKFAST & SNACKS
By Dr. Kerry Graff

Week 2- Game Plan. This week you are going to:

1. Enact your weekly plan for meal planning and shopping (this week you're shopping for 4Leaf breakfasts and snacks).
2. Start eating a 4Leaf breakfast every day.
3. Start eating only healthy snacks.
4. Keep track of your progress using the 4leaf Survey daily reporting version.
5. Toss or give away all of your unhealthy breakfast foods if you haven't already done so.
6. Start thinking about some 4Leaf lunch options for next week.
7. Start stocking your pantry with healthy staples (oats, nuts, beans, grains like bulgur, brown rice and quinoa, etc.)

BREAKFAST. Skipping breakfast denies your body the fuel it needs to get moving and sets you up for food cravings later in the day. SO DONT SKIP BREAKFAST! For most people, breakfast is what we call a routine meal, meaning we tend to eat almost the same thing every day.

It's essential that all *routine* meals are 4Leaf (80% or more of the calories come from whole plants). You have almost no chance to eat at a 4Leaf level overall if a meal that you eat almost every day is not 4Leaf.

You will need to find a 4Leaf breakfast that you like AND that will deliver enough calories so that you can make it to lunch without getting hungry. (Alternatively, you can plan a mid-morning healthy snack.) There are a million options, but below are a few of our favorites to get you started:

Sailors Daily Oatmeal
(what Jim Hicks eats just about every morning)

1. Start with any brand of oatmeal (*old fashioned, not quick cook*) that has only one ingredient--whole rolled (or steel cut) oats.

2. Put the oatmeal in a bowl along with a few raisins, add a few ounces of cold water and top off with unsweetened non-dairy milk. If you haven't tried oatmeal cold, you definitely should; and you may never eat hot oatmeal again.

3. While the oats soak, cut up a medley of your favorite fruit and put on top.

4. If you find yourself getting hungry before lunch, just add more oats to your breakfast. That should do the trick.

5. This meal can be prepared from start to finish in five minutes and can be eaten at any time of day or night. It's my go-to meal when I come home from a trip late at night.

Steel-cut oats and fruit
(what Kerry Graff eats just about every morning)

1.Put ½ cup of steel cut oats (2 servings worth) into a pot on the stove. Add 2 cups of water and turn on heat to medium.

2. While that is cooking, cut up and eat a half a grapefruit. If it is really delicious, eat the other half too.

3. Let the dog out, wash the dishes that didn't get done last night and stir the oats a few times.

4. Slice a banana into a big bowl and add the oats when they have finished cooking.

5. Add some blueberries. (I use frozen so they cool the oats off enough that I don't have to wait to eat it.)

6. Add a few walnuts, some cinnamon, and a splash of almond milk.

7. Eat until comfortably full. Usually I finish the whole thing.

OK, it is a little embarrassing how much I eat for breakfast. But seriously, if I don't eat this volume of food, I am hungry before lunch. And I still lost 25 pounds eating all this food and am now at a very healthy weight.

You hate oatmeal? My first response is to tell you to GET OVER IT, because oatmeal is seriously good for you. *Like a cholesterol sponge.* Well, that's not really how it works, but you get the idea. My second response is to ask if you have had the steel cut version, which has a firmer texture and nuttier taste. Usually, people's objection to food is related to texture and not taste, and the texture of steel cut oats is less, well, objectionable! But if you just can't stomach it…

Whole grain cereal is a decent option, although it is somewhat processed and you need to be sure there isn't added sugar. Add fruit, and make sure to use plant-based rather than cow's milk.

Fruit and/or veggie smoothie. There are a million versions of this. Below is my daughter's "go to" breakfast smoothie. It takes less than 2 minutes to make.

1.   Place ripe banana in blender.

2. Add a few frozen strawberries and/or blueberries.

3. Add a little maple syrup (optional, unless you are my daughter…)

4. Add just enough fruit juice or almond milk for the blender to blend everything together.

Potato and veggie scramble. This is obviously not quick to make, but it is my favorite Saturday morning breakfast. I even got my local diner to start making it for me if I'm out to breakfast with friends--thanks, Lafayette!

If you have leftover potatoes, use them. If not,

1. Wash and dice a potato into ½ inch pieces. Place in a bowl and cook in microwave on high for 3 minutes.

2. While that is cooking, cut up your veggies. Use any of the following or whatever you have on hand:

Sliced onion, asparagus, broccoli, tomatoes (fresh or sundried) spinach, peppers (any kind--I really like banana peppers) and mushrooms.

3. Place a skillet on medium heat and once hot, add the onions (if you are using) first. **You do not need any oil**! After these have cooked a bit, add the other veggies, starting with the potatoes, which should be soft by the time they come out of the microwave.

4. Then add the things that take longer to cook (like raw broccoli and asparagus) followed by the quicker cooking things (like peppers and spinach).

5. Add black olives if you wish. And some black pepper.

6. Serve. Consider topping it with hot sauce, salsa or hummus. Yum!

There a ton of options for breakfast foods. If none of the above appeal to you or if you need more variety, see Chapter 13 for recipe resources.

What about juice for breakfast? As mentioned earlier, since fruit or vegetable juice (whether packaged or fresh) is not a whole plant, it does not count as a serving of fruit or veggies on the 4Leaf Survey. It is missing the all-important fiber that makes your body run so efficiently and it also contains a concentrated load of sugar. For these reasons, we don't advise that you make fruit or vegetable juice a part of your daily routine.

What if I'm just not hungry in the morning? Eat at least a little fruit anyway and have some on hand for a mid-morning snack. If you don't eat breakfast, that donut at the office is going to be calling your name by mid-morning.

SNACKS. While you are getting used to how much you need to eat to get you to the next meal (you will need to eat significantly more volume now than you did before), you will need to have some healthy snacks on hand. Also, some people just can't comfortably eat enough whole, plant-based food at one sitting to provide sufficient calories to last them 5-6 hours until the next meal.

These folks will need to routinely add snacks into their daily routine. By snacks, I'm talking about quick-to-grab, ready-to-go foods that are just as healthy as the 4Leaf meals you are eating. So I'm not talking about crackers or potato chips. Some examples of easy-to-eat 4Leaf snacks you might have on hand:

- Bananas, apples, grapes or clementines

- Celery with a little peanut butter
- Cut up veggies and oil-free hummus
- Air popped popcorn

What about nuts? We do not recommend that you snack on nuts or seeds. Why? Because they average over 70% fat and if you are HUNGRY, you most likely will end up eating a lot of calories snacking on these. Fill up on something less calorie dense and save nuts and seeds to be used sparingly elsewhere, like sprinkled lightly on your oatmeal or salad.

APPENDIX E -- GOING 4LEAF SERIES
WEEK 3: LUNCH
By Dr. Kerry Graff

Week 3- Game Plan. This week you are going to:

1. Continue your plan for meal planning and shopping (this week you're shopping for breakfasts, snacks and now lunches)
2. Continue eating a 4Leaf breakfast every day.
3. Start batch cooking your lunches.
4. Start eating a 4Leaf lunch every day.
5. Continue eating healthy snacks.
6. Keep track of your progress using the 4Leaf Survey daily reporting version.
7. Start thinking about some 4Leaf dinner options for next week.
8. Continue stocking your pantry with healthy staples.
9. Buy some additional kitchen gadgets like a crockpot or blender if you feel that they would be helpful.

Lunch. For some of us, lunch is a routine meal and pretty similar from day to day. For others, this is not the case. If you like more variety at lunch than you do for breakfast, you will need to find multiple options for lunch that are 4Leaf. Whether or not you eat lunch at home or at the office, it is much easier to eat 4Leaf if you make it yourself!

We strongly recommend that you learn to cook in batches so that you ALWAYS have a 4Leaf meal ready to warm up for all those times when you don't feel like cooking or don't have time. That said, Jim and I have very different interpretations of "cooking in batches."

The Jim Hicks Way of "cooking in batches": Jim lives alone and doesn't have a lot of cooking experience, so if he can eat 4Leaf, you really have no excuse. He has a routine meal that he calls his *Sailors Daily Lunch (or Dinner)*. It basically includes a medley of grains and legumes that he cooks about once every two weeks. He then packages them in ten, one-serving plastic containers, putting eight of them in the freezer and the other two in the fridge. After using one or two from the fridge, he replaces them from the freezer; therefore, he always has the base of his go-to lunch ready to heat up quickly.

The remainder of the meal consists of vegetables or greens that he cooks slightly on top of the rice/beans as they are heated in the microwave. Finally, he adds an assortment of raw fruit and/or veggies on top. Although this regimen may sound boring, he insists that it is not and that he really looks forward to eating this meal every single time. Depending on season, the possible combinations are endless. His method depends on the fact that he has a microwave available. This works for him. It may or may not work for you.

You can also find his *Sailors Daily Lunch or Dinner* under Recipes at 4leafprogram.com

The Kerry Graff Way of "cooking in batches": I work fulltime and have kids, so my life is crazy busy. But I really love to cook and especially like to try out new recipes. So, every weekend I make a large pot of soup AND a large bean or grain-based salad that will last for several lunches. This allows me to have a 4Leaf meal ready quickly as I dart home from work for lunch and to let the dog out. I can also pack any of these to eat at work if I know I won't make it home for lunch, but my dog will be a bit desperate for her potty break. Here are a few of my "go to" lunches:

Black Bean and Corn Salad

- 1/3 cup fresh lime juice
- 1 clove garlic, minced
- 1 teaspoon salt
- 1/8 teaspoon red pepper flakes
- 2 (15oz) cans of black beans rinsed and drained
- 1 ½ cups frozen corn kernels, thawed
- 1 avocado-diced
- 1 red pepper, chopped
- 1 cup cherry tomatoes, cut in quarters
- 6 green onions, sliced thinly
- ¼ cup (or more) fresh cilantro

Mix lime juice, garlic, salt and red pepper flakes in a small jar.

In a large bowl, combine all the other ingredients. Pour the lime dressing over the salad and toss. Serve alone or over greens.

Tabouli Salad

- 1 cup of dry bulgar
- 1 lemon
- 1 large clove of garlic, minced
- 1 teaspoon dried mint
- ¾ teaspoon salt
- 4 green onions, sliced thinly
- 1 1/2 cups of cherry tomatoes, cut in quarters
- 1 cucumber, seeded and diced
- 1 (15oz) can of chickpeas, rinsed and drained
- A ton of chopped parsley--at least 1 large bunch

Boil 1 cup of water and pour over the bulgar to soak until soft (about 20 minutes). While this is soaking, juice the lemon and mix with the garlic, mint and salt. Chop up all the vegetables. Pour any residual water off the bulgar and add the lemon juice mixture. Add the veggies. Mix well. Chill and serve.

Quick Greens and Beans

- 1 large head of escarole, washed and chopped
- 2 cloves of garlic, minced
- 1 medium onion, chopped
- 6 cups of vegetable broth
- 1 (15oz) can of cannellini beans
- ½ teaspoon dried red pepper flakes
- Salt to taste

Heat a large pot over medium heat. Add the onion to the dry pot and stir for a minute or so until the onion starts to turn a little brown. Continue to sauté the onion in small amounts of vegetable broth until the onion starts to soften. Add the garlic and continue to sauté, adding just enough broth to keep it from sticking. When the onion is translucent, add the red pepper flakes, vegetable broth, beans and escarole. Cook for about 15 minutes. Add salt to taste.

Another of my favorite lunches is whole wheat pita bread stuffed with roasted red pepper hummus, sliced cucumber, tomatoes, black olives and spinach. I also always have on hand at home a few store-bought soups that are 4Leaf. Favorites are Amy's organic lentil vegetable soup and black bean soup.

If you have a Wegmans grocery store near you, and I sincerely hope that you do, they make three prepared soups that are 4Leaf, although they have more salt than I'd like—Moroccan Lentil Chickpea Soup, Black Bean Soup, and Vegetable Barley Soup. If the soup, sandwich and/or salad doesn't satisfy me, I'll end the meal with a sliced apple, topped with a tablespoon of organic peanut butter.

A word of caution: A big bowl of fruit or a big salad of vegetables is not a complete meal. Why not? Because it doesn't have enough calories to keep you going until your next meal. If you aren't eating enough to keep you satisfied, you will be tempted to eat junk. Don't go there! We recommend that you incorporate some starches in each meal: things like grains, legumes and potatoes (but not French fries or potato chips). Eat until you are comfortably full and always have healthy snacks available.

A final word about routine meals. We cannot overstress the importance of making sure that the meals you eat regularly are 4Leaf meals. If you can't master those routine meals, it will be nearly impossible to reach the 4Leaf level of eating.

IMPORTANT. By the end of Week 3, get rid of ALL your remaining contraband.

APPENDIX F -- GOING 4LEAF SERIES
WEEK 4: DINNER
By Dr. Kerry Graff

Week 4- Game Plan. This week you are going to:

1. Continue your plan for shopping and meal planning. (now you're shopping for breakfast, lunch, snacks, AND dinner)
2. Batch cook at least some of your lunches and dinners.
3. Continue eating your 4Leaf breakfast.
4. Continue eating your 4Leaf lunch.
5. Continue eating your healthy snacks.
6. Start eating a 4Leaf dinner.
7. Keep track of your progress using the 4Leaf Survey daily reporting version.
8. Get rid of the rest of the unhealthy foods in the house, if you haven't already.

Dinner is not usually a routine meal, meaning that a great many people typically have something different most days of the week at dinner time. That doesn't necessarily mean that it is harder to make dinner a 4Leaf meal, just that you will need to do more planning, unless you are like Jim, who is lucky enough to eat out almost every night!

See his Chapter 15 on eating 4Leaf outside the home. For the times he eats at home, he just has one of his *Sailors Daily* meals. Us "normal" folks, who don't eat out most nights of the week, need a workable plan for eating 4Leaf evening meals at home.

This is where you need to spend a little time on your planning day, picking out what you are going to eat for the week. You don't need to map out what food you plan to eat on which day (although you can be that specific if you want to) but a general plan of what meals you will be making and when you have time to make them is important.

Like I said previously, I typically do a lot of my cooking on the weekend. In addition to the multi-day supply of soup and the grain or bean-based salad I prepare for lunches during the week, I usually also make something for dinner on Saturday and/or Sunday that will give me leftovers to eat during the week. I know that I will have no time to cook on Tuesday and Thursday—these are always "heat-up-something-I've-already-made" days.

Mondays and Wednesdays I get home with a little time to cook, so I need recipes for those days that will not take a ton of time. Friday is either leftovers or dinner out, usually at a Japanese restaurant (that my son loves) that makes a delicious vegetable teriyaki.

So, KNOW YOUR SCHEDULE and make a plan that fits your week.

This was my dinner schedule this past week:

Saturday—Dinner out with the kids. Had tomato soup to start and then whole grains with veggies. The grains were supposed to have steak over them but I had them serve it without the meat ("Tiger Shrimp, Hold the Shrimp" technique--See Chapter 15).

Sunday—Black bean and sweet potato enchiladas. This is a time intensive recipe at 90 minutes BUT usually this would give me two days worth of leftovers, so it's really only 30 minutes of prep per meal. This day, however, I had friends over for dinner AND sent them home with some enchiladas, so I only had a day's worth left.

Monday—Thai coconut soup--took 35 minutes to make, start to finish.

Tuesday—Left over enchiladas

Wednesday— Vegetable stir-fry with brown rice

Thursday—Left over Thai soup

Friday—Left over tabouli (from my lunches) in whole wheat pita pockets with roasted red pepper hummus. Apple with peanut butter for dessert. And a beer.

There are way too many options for dinners to list them here. For a lot more ideas, check out all the resources in Chapter 13 (page 45) entitled: Recipes Are Everywhere.

APPENDIX G—AN EXERCISE ROUTINE THAT WORKS FOR ME

By J. Morris Hicks

Ideally, you'll have the kind of schedule and budget that permits you to join a fitness center and hire a personal trainer to get you started--and keep you going. But not everyone has that luxury. Here's the way I do it:

- Visiting the fitness center in my building EVERY day that I wake up in my Stamford, CT, home-- varying my schedule, but always including both aerobic and strength training.

- Taking a brisk 40-minute walk every day that weather permits. (This used to be a run, until my son told me to shift to a brisk walk after hearing me complaining about my knees.)

- Engaging in sports and recreation activities that keep my body in motion: skiing, golfing, sailing, cycling and walking. (I quit tennis after rupturing my Achilles tendon in 2010.)

- Walking to the grocery or to my New York train from my Connecticut residence and walking or taking the subway (lots of steps) when in the city.

- Not always searching for the closest parking spot and developing a habit of frequently taking the stairs.

My recommendation is that you do a little research, chart your course and get moving--with this word of caution from Dr. Graff: "Although just about everyone would benefit from professional advice on this extremely important topic, it is very important that you get that advice if you have significant medical issues or have been very inactive for a long time."

A WORD ABOUT FOOTNOTES

You may have noticed that there are no footnotes in this 4Leaf Guide. In an attempt to make this information more accessible to the average reader, the authors acknowledge critical sources in the body of the book where appropriate. Additionally, much of what is written comes from the authors' personal experiences.

In his earlier book, *Healthy Eating, Healthy World*, (BenBella 2011), Jim provided 306 footnotes as he meticulously documented all that he had learned in his 10,000 hours of study on the multi-faceted, "big picture" consequences of our food choices. It is a great next read if you are interested in learning more about the background of what is presented in this 4Leaf Guide.

While writing that 2011 book, Jim realized that there needed to be a better and simpler way to communicate the optimal diet for humans without using the word vegan, which has negative connotations for many and doesn't convey that "whole" plant-based foods are critical for health. That's why he created the 4Leaf concept in 2009, and it was that concept that caught the attention of Dr. Kerry Graff as she searched the internet for handy tools to help her communicate healthy eating to her patients.

There was one thing missing from those 4Leaf materials at that time: a handy guide-book to help patients not only understand why the whole food, plant-based diet is so crucial to human and environmental health, but also how to actually transition to eating this way. The authors are thrilled to have created such a book and even more thrilled that you are now holding it in your hands.

ABOUT THE AUTHORS

Dr. Kerry Graff began laying the foundation for her medical career at Cornell, graduating summa cum laude as a biology major in 1990. After graduating from the University of Pittsburgh School of Medicine cum laude four years later, she completed a three-year Family Practice Residency at UPMC Shadyside in Pittsburgh. In 1997, she relocated to Canandaigua, NY, where she was employed by Thompson Health for the next nine years, providing primary care, including obstetrics.

In 2006, she opened her own practice that allowed her more flexibility in the way she practiced medicine. Then, after watching the powerful documentary, "Forks Over Knives" in 2013, she adopted a whole food, plant-based diet herself and quickly began experiencing a host of huge improvements in her health. She knew immediately that her medical career was about to change in a big way.

So it was back to Cornell, where she quickly earned her Certificate in Plant-Based Nutrition from eCornell and the T. Colin Campbell Center for Nutrition Studies and began incorporating the 4Leaf Survey as a teaching tool in her medical practice to help patients transition to a healthier diet. She reports that the results have been absolutely amazing, and that the 4Leaf Program has become an integral part of the way she practices medicine today. She currently serves as Chief Medical Officer at 4Leaf Global, LLC, helping to create teaching tools for patients.

J. Morris Hicks is the author of *Healthy Eating, Healthy World* and the creator of the 4Leaf concept. Shortly after learning all about the many alarming truths regarding our food choices in 2003, Jim realized that there needed to be a better way to explain healthy eating to the world. The "V" words, at best, convey more information about what you're avoiding than what you ARE eating. He began developing the 4Leaf concept in 2009 and introduced it to the public in his 2011 book, co-authored with his son, Jason.

A former strategic management consultant and later, a senior corporate executive with Ralph Lauren in New York, Jim has always focused on the "big picture" when analyzing any issue. In 2002, after becoming curious about the "optimal diet" for humans, he began a study of what we eat from a global perspective--discovering many startling issues and opportunities along the way.

In addition to a BS in Industrial Engineering from Auburn University and an MBA from the University of Hawaii, he holds a Certificate in Plant-Based Nutrition from eCornell and the T. Colin Campbell Center for Nutrition Studies, where he has also been a member of the board of directors since 2012.

Having concluded that our food choices hold the key to the sustainability of our civilization, he has made them his #1 priority--exploring all avenues for influencing humans everywhere to move back to the natural, plant-based diet for our species--in the interest of promoting health, hope and harmony on planet Earth.

This book contains about 44,000 words. By comparison, since 2011, J. Morris Hicks has published 900-plus articles and over one million words relative to this crucial global topic on his website at hpjmh.com.

Susan Benigas

Founder of The Plantrician Project, Co-Founder of the
International Plant-Based Healthcare Conference
(pbnhc.com) and Executive Director of The American
College of Lifestyle Medicine

A DOCTOR'S WORD
IS SECOND ONLY TO GOD'S

In 2005, I was a featured speaker at the Missouri
Foundation for Health Obesity Summit, sharing the stage
with then Arkansas Governor Mike Huckabee. In his
opening remarks, he told about being in the 4th grade in
Arkansas when his teacher asked the students to bring in
symbols of their religion for show and tell.

One of Mike's classmates was Jewish, so he brought in a
Menorah and explained its significance. Another little girl
was Catholic and brought her special Rosary for all to
see. Ten-year-old Mike Huckabee told his class that he was
Southern Baptist and came toting a covered casserole dish
as a symbol of his religion and its abundance of food
related fellowship!

Needless to say, the audience roared with laughter. The
Governor chuckled, as well, but went on to explain the sad
reality of our prevailing health statistics, noting that regular
church-attendees have higher obesity and chronic disease
rates than non-church-goers.

Fast forward ten years, and we're in worse shape now than
we were back in 2005; yet, the good news is that up to

80% of all healthcare spending is tied the treatment of conditions resulting from poor lifestyle choices. And, as you've read throughout this book, food trumps all.

Over the past few years, I've come to recognize that the #1 cause of most chronic disease AND the #1 cause of many of our most pressing global sustainability issues is one and the same: our western industrialized diet. The foods we should be eating to protect our health and prevent disease are the exact same choices we should make in regard to the big picture of global sustainability, natural resource preservation, and our ability to feed the world's burgeoning population.

From a Judeo Christian perspective, it's truly remarkable that that which God designed to be the foundation for man's food is what's best for our health and for our planet.

"I give you every seed-bearing plant on the face of the whole earth and every tree that has fruit with seed in it. They will be yours for food." –Genesis 1:29

I'm always the one telling Jim that I'd prefer he stop referring to humans as "the infestation of planet earth." He does have a point in that we humans have run roughshod over the earth, particularly during the past century. We were entrusted with this beautiful planet and all of its natural resources, yet we have been horrible stewards---of the Earth and of our own health.

Even Pope Francis is becoming a leading voice in raising awareness about global sustainability, although he has yet to acknowledge the powerful connection to our food choices. I believe he simply does not yet know what he does not know. He soon will if J. Morris Hicks has anything to do with it.

Jim Hicks and I first crossed paths in early 2008, both recently having had our paradigm-shifts, which Jim refers to as his "blinding flash of the obvious." We have been close friends, colleagues and collaborators ever since, bonded by our shared passion for the subject matter outlined in this book.

In 2013, I co-founded *The Plantrician Project*, a not-for-profit dedicated to creating events, tools and resources for medical professionals and their patients and clients. Together with Dr. Scott Stoll and Tom Dunnam, both introduced to me by Jim, we produce the CME-accredited International Plant-based Nutrition Healthcare Conference (pbnhc.com) each year and the International Cardiovascular Nutrition Summit. We also provide plantbaseddocs.com as mentioned earlier.

The impetus for *Plantrician* was this burning question: "How do we most effectively reach, inspire and guide all people of the western world and emerging economies in making the shift from the SAD to the predominantly whole food, plant-based dietary lifestyle that is optimal for human health, healthcare system sustainability and global resource preservation?"

Physicians and healthcare professionals hold the key—as they're the most-trusted source of patient and client dietary recommendations. Individuals may read books and watch films that espouse the benefits of a plant-based lifestyle; but, until physicians and other wellness practitioners understand and embrace the benefits and, in turn, promote patient adoption, this dietary shift on a broad scale will be elusive. Yet, our medical education system is nearly devoid of nutrition education, focusing almost exclusively on an allopathic, "diagnose, treat and medicate" curriculum.

It's organizations like *The Plantrician Project* that are leading the charge—shining a bright light on the need for our clinicians and allied health professionals to learn about and embrace the overwhelming evidence that supports the efficacy of whole, plant-based nutrition and its ability to prevent, suspend and often, even reverse the chronic, degenerative disease that's wreaking havoc on hundreds of millions of lives and entire nations around the world.

Prior to meeting Jim, I had been president of a worksite health promotion company, taking the status quo approach: biometric screenings and health risk assessments, with employees found to have chronic conditions being directed to see their primary care physicians and get a script. This was followed by the drum beat of medication persistency. I finally took a step back and asked myself, "Did God really design us all to become chronically ill and dependent on prescription meds?"

I was also beginning to question why so little effort and funding was dedicated to identifying and eradicating the cause of disease. While "prevention" was given lip service, it was usually in the context of mammograms or colonoscopies. Prevention and early detection are not synonymous. Far from it!

It was perfect timing when I was invited to a presentation by a local oncologist. She began her talk by sharing the story about her previous ill health issues; including arthritis, fibromyalgia, and a skin condition. She said that she had been surviving on caffeinated beverages and the treats her patients brought to her. She proceeded to hold up a book and say, "This book has changed my life and is changing the lives of many of my patients."

It was *The China Study* by T. Colin Campbell. I bought a copy and could not put it down, now referring to it as the most paradigm-shifting read of my adult life. Not only was it the most comprehensive study of the correlation between nutrition and human health ever published, it also connected the dots between the status quo and our broken disease and disability care system.

I finally understood that we do not have a "health" care system, but, rather, a system so aptly described by medical journalist Shannon Brownlee in *Escape Fire*, "We have a disease care system, and we have a *very profitable* disease care system—it doesn't want you to die and it doesn't want you to get well; it just wants you to keep coming back for the care of your chronic disease."

The winds of change are blowing, as physicians and medical professionals around the world awaken to the fact that a pill for every ill is not sustainable, nor is it in the best interest of patients.

Dr. Kerry Graff, whom I had the pleasure of meeting at Lifestyle Medicine 2014, is a glowing example of a physician who is re-engineering her practice in a way that enables her to educate, equip and empower her patients with the information and resources needed for them to seize an enormous amount of control over their health.

Using food as medicine must become the foundation of a transformed and sustainable healthcare system, ushering in *sustainable* human health and a *sustainable* world. This information-packed 4Leaf Guide is just what the doctor ordered--providing a powerful tool that medical professionals can use to confidently prescribe the 4Leaf lifestyle to their patients and clients.

For more information or to contact us, visit:
4leafprogram.com

Take the 4Leaf Survey at:
4leafsurvey.com

For hundreds of articles relevant to topics covered in this book, visit the website of J. Morris Hicks at:
hpjmh.com

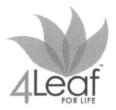

A refreshing dose of clarity in a confusing world

CAUTION. Eating the 4Leaf way (described throughout this book) may quickly decrease your need for medications. You should tell your physician what you're doing. If he/she is not familiar with, or skeptical of, this eating style, please direct him or her to plantrician.org and nutritionstudies.org.